Coping With Caregiving

A Common-Sense Approach
to Home Care

Coping With Caregiving

A Common-Sense Approach to Home Care

By Inez Pirie, RN (ret.)

Ruhl Press
Amarillo, Texas

Coping With Caregiving

COPING WITH CAREGIVING: A COMMON-SENSE APPROACH TO HOME CARE is an original publication of Ruhl Press.

Copyright © 1996 by Inez Pirie
Published by arrangement with the author
Library of Congress Catalogue Number LCCN 96-092061
ISBN: 0-9650215-0-5

Publisher's Cataloging in Publication
(Prepared by Quality Books Inc.)

Pirie, Inez.
  Coping with caregiving: a common-sense guide to home care/ Inez Pirie.
  p. cm.
  Includes bibliographical references and index.
  ISBN 0-9650215-0-5

  1. Home nursing.   2. Care of the sick.   3. Caregivers.   I. Title.

RT61.P57 1996   649.8
                                           QBI96-20020

First Ruhl Press Printing: March 1996

Quantity discounts are available on bulk purchases of this book for workshops, fund raising or gift giving. Special booklets can be created to fit your special needs. For information contact Ruhl Press, P.O. Box 8100-153, Amarillo, Texas 79114, Phone or Fax 1-806-354-8248.

BEEPER (806) 354-8212

Acknowledgements

I would like to thank the many caregivers and friends who shared their thoughts and experiences in caregiving. From these discussions came many practical suggestions and solutions.

A special thanks to my editor, Geraldine McBride, for her understanding, valuable suggestions and expertise, to Margaret Louthan for her encouragement, and to Sherri Morrison, who captured the essence of caregiving in her cover design.

Most of all I want to thank my husband, Bill Pirie, whose encouragement and suggestions were exactly what I needed. For one who is never ill and who has never had long-term caregiving responsibilities, his instinctive understanding and objective viewpoint generated the astute questions that made me consider or justify my answers. His fingerprints are on this book also.

This book is dedicated to the caring, responsible person
who provides care for one who cannot survive alone.

To my daughters, Rae and Sherri, and their families

In memory of my Quaker parents and
a son who fought with quiet courage.

Table of Contents

Table of Contents

Coping With Caregiving

Finding a pronoun for "your disabled love one" has been difficult. I have decided to use "he" when generically referring to the patient and "she" when speaking of you, the caregiver. This makes for easier reading and better continuity.

About The Author

The author, Inez Ruhl Pirie, is a registered nurse who has retired after an active and varied nursing career. She has been an Instructor in professional schools of nursing, a Nursing Director (administrator) in hospitals and extended care facilities, a Disaster Nursing Supervisor for the National Red Cross in disaster situations, and a Director of Nursing Programs in a community agency.

During her nursing career, Pirie has provided care for chronically ill, disabled and elderly patients. Some of those discharged from the hospital were readmitted a short time later. If she found the patient depressed and dehydrated and the caregiver exhausted and discouraged, she wondered if the nurses could have better prepared both the patient and his caregiver for the problems to be faced at home.

Her concerns were reinforced when her young son was diagnosed with Hodgkin's Disease and she waited with other caregivers at cancer research and treatment centers. During the years his disease was in and out of remission, she shared the concerns and unspoken sadness of fellow caregivers. She recognized that inexperienced caregivers courageously struggle to meet their loved one's needs.

It was from these experiences and her efforts to help caregivers that the book was born. Pirie believes that it is not the basic caregiving skills that are the problem, for everyone has learned how to give baths, make beds and fix food. It is the debilitating effects of a prolonged illness and the side effects of treatment that leave the caregiver questioning how to provide good care.

The author has not written an "everything-you-want-to-know" book, but a quick reference for caregivers to locate many answers. She supplies a common-sense approach to solutions. She also defines the responsibilities and limits of the caregiving role. The reader will find suggestions for ending conflicts and planning free time for herself. It is a supportive tool which makes caregiving easier.

A Word About
The Tips And Shortcuts Of Caregiving

This book, *Coping With Caregiving*, is a "survival kit" for anyone who helps care for a disabled, elderly or chronically-ill loved one at home.

As a nurse, I have listened to concerned caregivers as they readmitted a chronically-ill loved one to the hospital, as we sat together during their loved one's chemotherapy treatments and as they made arrangements for a nursing home admission. These inexperienced, exhausted relatives or friends had provided daily care at home, and would question how well they had met their disabled loved one's needs.

Whatever the situation, the circumstances were similar. The caregivers had often tried to make decisions based on a poor understanding of fragmented information. The medical terms were unfamiliar. Explanations were brief. Given the stress of the situation, new information often made little sense to them. They felt ill-prepared to meet a loved one's changing needs. They needed a "survival kit" with discussions of various conditions, easy instructions for general care and descriptions of possible complications to watch for.

If you are a caregiver and share your life with someone who is unable to survive alone, this book can help. It was created from the needs and past experiences of nurses and others. The book stresses the "how's" and "why's" of caregiving, offers ways for those involved to live more comfortably together and discusses the difficult decisions that you, as a caregiver, may be forced to make. You will find help when you can no longer manage alone or when your loved one's life is ending.

The book does not discuss the basic caregiving skills people acquire as they rear their family, but builds on those basic skills. You will discover how to use shortcuts, avoid problems, watch for complications and report to the doctor. You should feel comfortable in your caregiver role as you understand how to cope with the pressures of confinement and decision making.

By looking at the page of contents, you will realize that this is a "how to" book, a quick reference for help with a problem situation. I have

A Word About The Tips and Shortcuts of Caregiving

included the most common, time-consuming and frustrating problems faced by many caregivers. The text contains subtle reminders of your right to ask questions and will help you identify the choices available. It describes how to help your disabled loved one make an informed decision.

As I write, I consider this book to be a discussion between us: you, the involved caregiver, and me, as we share our cups of coffee. I hope you find the information of value, and I would be very interested to learn how well it has met your needs.

The book was written with care - for I have walked in your shoes.

LISTEN

When I ask you to listen to me
and you start giving advice,
you have not done what I asked.

When I ask you to listen to me
and you begin to tell me why I shouldn't feel that way,
you are trampling on my feelings.

When I ask you to listen to me
and you feel you have to do something to solve my problem,
you have failed me, strange as it may seem.

Listen! All I asked was that you listen....
not talk or do....just hear me.
When you do something for me that I can and need to do
for myself, you contribute to my fear and weakness.
And I can do for myself; I'm not helpless
Maybe discouraged and faltering, but not helpless.

When you accept as a simple fact that I do feel what I feel,
no matter how irrational, then I can quit trying to convince
you and can get about the business of understanding what's
behind this irrational feeling.
And when that's clear, the answers are obvious and I
don't need your advice.
Irrational feelings make sense when we understand what's
behind them.
So please listen and just hear me. And if you want to talk, wait a
minute for your turn; and I'll listen to you.

....Anonymous....

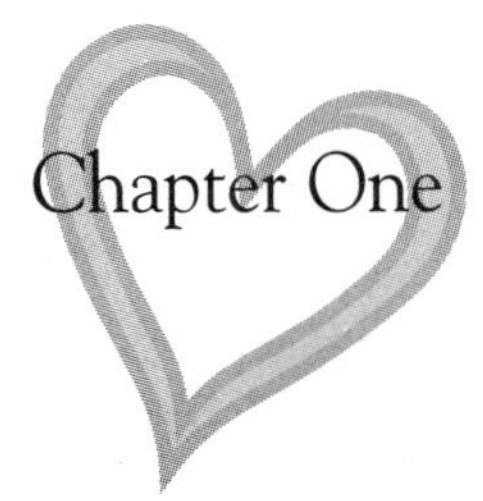

Chapter One

CARING FOR
THE CAREGIVER

The person who has agreed to provide care for someone has assumed an ongoing responsibility. The caregiver devotes time to the needs of another as she ignores the extra hours, frequent exhaustion and loss of personal freedom. Eventually, despite the urgent needs of a disabled loved one, she must place a priority on her own needs. Her physical health, mental stability and general well-being must be protected.

Who cares for someone when they can no longer survive alone - a concerned, involved caregiver.

You may be a wife, daughter or daughter-in-law, so everyone agrees that you are the logical one to become the primary caregiver. In rarer cases, you may be a husband, son, relative or friend. You have volunteered or have accepted the role by default, since others have demanding jobs, children to rear, live at a distance or are in poor health. Whether your commitment is short-term or an ongoing responsibility, you are the compassionate person who listens, reassures and spends time with a lonely loved one.

As days go by, you may accept that you are the only one responsible for the day-to-day care of your loved one. Searching for a relief caregiver, if not the first rule of caregiving, should certainly receive a high priority.

Where do you find someone to provide relief for a few hours, a day or overnight? You may ask relatives to provide respite care. They may have been waiting for your call or you may hear apologies, such as they would help but do not have the time or they realize that they cannot provide the care you do. It is the dependable, unselfish family member or friend who offers a few hours respite care on a weekly basis that earns your heartfelt gratitude.

If you have had little support or dependable relief from others, check the phone book for community agencies. Locate the responsible person in local church groups and ask if they will provide a sitter for a few hours. Community organizations may offer transportation to treatment centers, doctors' offices or community centers plus other services. A home health agency offers care for a fee. It has a staff who will provide personal care, perform housekeeping and cooking chores, or give more skilled nursing care. The hourly charge varies according to the skills required. A qualified nurse will evaluate your loved one's needs before selecting a dependable staff member to serve as relief caregiver.

Contact friends and try word of mouth to help locate relief caregivers. One family employed a retired nurse to care for their mother, bedfast from Alzheimer's, while they were at work. Another family located two sisters who were experienced home caregivers. They agreed to divide around-the-clock care so that an elderly couple could remain at home. Weekend relief care was provided by the son and daughter-in-law. The total cost for care was far less than nursing home care.

The caregivers I have known are often physically and mentally exhausted. Caregiving has become the focal point of their days. When their "patient" becomes increasingly debilitated and requires more professional care, the decision to move him is a difficult one. Making the final decision to move the person into a nursing home may arouse a sense of guilt and may become as painful for the devoted caregiver as it is for the disabled.

Taking Care of Yourself

Now that you are a daily caregiver, you should make your job as easy as possible. Good caregiving is based on common sense, a lifetime of experience and an understanding of the special care needed for a specific condition. The knowledge you gain helps you become a more capable caregiver with time for yourself. It is up to you to plan for time to pursue your own interests. If you become ill or incapacitated, the disabled one still needs the same daily care. Caring for yourself protects both of you.

Tips for Self Protection:

- Stress may deplete the body's resources, so take a good vitamin and mineral supplement. Eat several small meals during the day to maintain energy.

- Stretch, deep breathe, and relax. Exercise a few minutes before getting out of bed in the morning and just before going to sleep at night.

- Be kind to your skin and kidneys by drinking liquids throughout the day. Try using herb mixes instead of salt to season food.

- Be aware of any noticeable gain or loss of weight. Are you eating extra sweets for quick energy or do you forget to eat when you are tired or worried?

- Protect your back. Learn to lift and push correctly. Most back injuries are one's own fault.

- Get enough rest. Take 30-45 minute naps during the day, especially when sleep has been interrupted at night. Exhaustion may lead to accidents and injuries.

- Don't ignore a physical or emotional problem - one often affects the other.

---

*The emphasis today is on preventive medicine,
which is based on a person's understanding
of wellness and how to help prevent illnesses.*

Stress can increase a borderline cholesterol level, elevate blood pressure and place a burden on the heart and other vital organs. It may cause you to be irritable and to feel exhausted. Consider your health in general. Make and keep doctors' appointments and describe any problems as accurately as possible. You may not be able to eliminate the stress from your busy life, but you can control and reduce it.

Several home tests are available that can help you evaluate your general health. These inexpensive tests are found in pharmacies, drugstores and large discount stores. Edward R. Pickney, MD, in his book, *Do it Yourself Medical Testing*, explains that before home tests can be marketed to consumers, the manufacturer must show that they are safe, at least 95% effective, and have been approved by the FDA. If you are in good health and symptom free, you may use home tests to help screen yourself. However, if symptoms develop suddenly, do not start self testing. See your physician as soon as possible. Some of the tests available are: a self-inflating blood pressure unit, a test for a urinary tract infection, assorted blood sugar tests, a test for occult blood in the stool and a test for cholesterol levels.

Suggestions to Help Maintain
A Stable Emotional Balance

- Start the day in a serene mood. Discover what works for you. Have a little faith that good things will happen despite the unexpected trials of life.

- When life gets hectic, take a break. Even the bathroom provides privacy and an opportunity for quiet moments.

- Recognize what you cannot change. You have choices. Change what needs to be changed - if you can.

- Share a few minutes with people who care about you. Call your friends and family. Don't let your life grow barren and empty. You must be a friend to keep friends.

- Laughter is healing, so bring more of it into your loved one's isolated world. Life can become a burden if you don't laugh at the funny, ridiculous and absurd things that happen.

- Show your love and kindness every day. Give your loved one hugs - he may receive very few. Remind him how important he is to you and others.

- Develop a forgiving attitude toward those you dislike. Wipe out old hurts and other burdensome "baggage" from yesterday. Forgive for your sake. You can protect yourself from any mistreatment in the future.

- We are the builders of the world we live in. If the one you and your loved one inhabit is a miserable place, change it. When one person changes the way he or she reacts toward a difficult situation, and acts differently, the situation changes. While we do not control another's tongue or actions, we control our own. We have more control and influence than we think we do.

- Give your loved one and yourself a break from each other - a respite. Make arrangements for a few hours of relief and free time each week. You can maintain your separate activities and your loved one will enjoy the break from daily routine.

When life gets hectic, try these "stress relievers":

- Wash the car.
- Pound a pillow.
- Dig in the earth.
- Paint an ugly table.
- Lie on the floor with your feet in a chair.
- Have your hair done and sleep under the dryer.
- Sing with gusto as you drive to the store. Ignore other's looks.
- Toss ice cream, fruit and juice in a blender - and share.
- Hug the cat, a grandchild, a neighbor or your disabled loved one.
- Take a hot shower, wrap up in a robe or comforter, lie down and turn on soft music. Close your eyes and remember a happy occasion. Remain quiet until you feel yourself relax.

Finally, I give you two caregiver's rules to live by:

Live in the present. Each sunrise you are given a new day with choices as to how to fill the hours. After care and attention to your disabled loved one, the time remaining is yours. This day will never come again - so don't waste today's opportunities, spend energy over yesterday's hurts or worry about an unknown tomorrow.

Give and receive help. Experienced caregivers who have faced similar crises will understand your problems, will appreciate your efforts and, if asked, will offer information and suggestions. Their support and patience may help you keep your life in balance and dispel the feeling that you are struggling alone. Others who have coped with similar situations may be found in support groups, church organizations, hospice programs and elsewhere.

Chapter Two

THE DOCTOR-PATIENT-CAREGIVER RELATIONSHIP

T he caregiver needs a direct line to the doctor who prescribes care. Without interfering with the special relationship between the doctor and his patient, she should be informed and understand the expected results of treatment. She should learn how to recognize and help prevent complications, and should feel free to ask advice. This chapter explains how to build a cooperative relationship.

The doctor-patient relationship, with easy communication and mutual trust, is a unique and private one. A caregiver or other family member will be given explanations and support; but he or she does not become an integral part of the relationship until the patient can no longer function in decision making. This is the relationship each of us want and expect to have with our physician.

A caregiver who is informed, observant and tactful becomes a valuable asset to the relationship. The good caregiver is a "home nurse" who notices day-to-day changes in the loved one's condition and can accurately report her observations to the doctor. The patient or the doctor may be unaware of these changes. To form a strong doctor-caregiver relationship, the caregiver should resist the inclination to diagnose or interpret symptoms. She should practice the three C's: remain calm, be concise, and be cooperative.

Your disabled loved one deserves your cooperative attitude toward his doctor. You need to be informed by the doctor of possible reactions to treatment and the early symptoms of unexpected complications. When the doctor trusts your observations and is accessible to you, you may be saved from needless anxiety and misunderstanding. You both share a common goal.

Through the years, the role of caregiver has changed. In years past, your great grandmother may have fought the battle for survival with herbs and home remedies. Despite her efforts, she lost loved ones to catastrophic illnesses, and her children were exposed to illness and death. Families are no longer exposed to the same struggles, and we often have unrealistic expectations for quick, dramatic cures. Patients frequently bestow the almost God-like qualities of "healer" on their doctor and relinquish responsibility for their own health. They forget that doctors are human and that researchers still search for cures. As a society, we have become distrustful if our recovery is slow or limited and may decide that the doctor failed, not us.

The doctor, too often, meets a poorly informed patient who presents a sketchy medical history, makes little effort to understand the doctor's explanations, skips doses of a medication and fails to keep scheduled appointments. The patient places himself in the doctor's hands, but "the healer" receives little help.

Authors Siegler and Osmons in their book *Patienthood* have labeled us "novices," who must quickly learn how to become responsible patients if we are to receive the best possible care - while maintaining our dignity and self respect. Today the emphasis is on maintaining good health habits and to better understand our bodies.

I suspect the doctor who practices medicine today prefers the inquisitive, determined and more responsible patient. The ill person may ask for explanations and take the time to consider his choices. Some doctors feel comfortable when confronted by a questioning, outspoken patient. Others do not. All doctors are pleased that once committed, their patient follows directions, reports any complications and discusses realistically his chances for recovery. He may gain more recovery than expected. No longer the "novice," the patient believes that he or she has entered a partnership with the doctor toward a future recovery.

You, as caregiver, have accepted certain responsibilities and the doctor needs to be aware of this fact. You should find ways to demonstrate that you can be a reasonable, cooperative member of the team without interfering with the doctor-patient relationship. If you are not acquainted with the doctor, you should:

- Call the doctor's office and ask for a short appointment.

- Briefly explain to the doctor how involved you are in your disabled loved one's care and mention your past experience.

- Explain your concerns about the patient's condition and ask questions about the care needed. Write your questions down before your visit.

- As you thank the doctor, assure him or her that you will try to be a well-informed, dependable helper who will report accurately.

Some doctors will charge for a "get acquainted" meeting.

The doctor has met you and had the opportunity to evaluate your involvement and stability. Remember that a good working relationship is an ongoing process. To be a well-informed member of the team, you should:

- Know the names of all medications ordered, the expected results and the possible side effects. Ask the pharmacist for help.

- Be able to give a brief medical history on the person.

- Contact the doctor's office and speak with the nurse if you have not understood the doctor's instructions or explanations.

- Before you call the doctor about a problem, review the sequence of events leading up to it (when started, what was done, etc.). The doctor will need an accurate description of symptoms:
    - Describe the problem and any noticeable changes.
    - Describe the type and location of pain (burning, throbbing, cutting, etc.).
    - Report vital signs. Take the temperature, pulse, and the blood pressure if the person feels weak or has a headache.

> —Report other details. For instance: "vomited three times during the last two hours," "is short of breath," "seems confused," etc.

Note: The nurse may ask for details of the problem before speaking to the doctor. She needs a brief report of your loved one's condition.

With few exceptions, a concerned doctor will welcome your assistance and will keep you informed of your loved one's present condition, the changes made in medications or treatments and the expected results. The doctor should take a moment to explain the kind of feedback he needs. If you have difficulty establishing a working relationship with the doctor or are concerned with your loved one's progress, you may:

- **Ask the doctor for more explanations.**

  Write your questions down, listen carefully and discuss his answers. Voice your concerns. Don't return home with unanswered questions. One lady, whose doctor had given few explanations during her office visits, asked for a final word before leaving. She asked,

  "If I become very ill, would you talk to me and explain what is happening?"

  The busy doctor seemed surprised, sat down and asked what was worrying her. He explained that he welcomed questions and would keep her better informed.

- **Ask for a second opinion.**

  Suggest to your loved one that a second opinion may give both of you greater peace of mind. The patient may ask for a referral or he may call a doctor of his choosing. You may assume this responsibility if he is incapable of responsible decision making. Ask that the most recent medical records be sent to the second doctor. You may be asked to sign a release. Your loved one has not switched doctors, just asked for another opinion.

- **Speak with the doctor's nurse or the pharmacist if side effects are upsetting or persist.**

  Many side effects will disappear within a few days, but should be reported. Some drugs will have a cumulative effect and need time to reach a therapeutic level. Do not stop the medicine without contacting the doctor for instructions. In one case, a chronic condition gave the person much misery until the medication was adjusted and had time to affect the muscle tone. After almost two weeks the condition suddenly cleared up.

Note: The patient benefits when he and the doctor have a history together. He is less well-served by changing doctors frequently, for each new doctor must become acquainted with his past medical history.

Having said that, your loved one may have legitimate reasons to consider transferring to another doctor, such as a lack of trust, poor communication or the doctor's inaccessibility.

- Ask another doctor if he will accept your loved one as a patient. (Your loved one should ask himself, if able). If so, inform the previous doctor's office. A release must be signed before a copy of all medical records, including a summary of X-ray findings, will be sent to the new doctor.

Patients have a right to be informed about their condition, the treatment being ordered, possible side effects to watch for, how medicines should be taken and the expected results. They should not hesitate to speak with the nurse in the doctor's office if they have unexpected symptoms or do not seem to be improving.

In the unwritten agreement between doctor and patient, the patient trusts the doctor to provide expert treatment, and the patient agrees to follow orders and try to get well.

Chapter Three

CARING FOR A DISABLED LOVED ONE

Most of us have had experience with basic caregiving as we reared our families. Besides such typical tasks of bathing or hair washing, care of a disabled loved one also includes monitoring elimination, skin breakdown and pain. This chapter will help you build on your past experiences with tips and suggestions for easier and faster daily caregiving. You will learn how problems and complications can be identified and prevented.

Planning Daily Care

A daily routine of personal care seems effortless as one considers the coming day's activities. The person who is disabled, weak or poorly-coordinated may find these same tasks time consuming and exhausting. At what point is your help needed?

Take the time to determine how much your loved one can do alone. You should offer help, but preserve his dignity and independence by permitting him to do as much as he is able. Evaluate his ability, and don't let him struggle until in frustration, he feels helpless.

You need a flexible plan for care if you want to bring a semblance of order to your days. Start by considering the person's established routine and keeping it. For instance: Monday and Friday are bath days with a bed change on Monday; after the daily nap is a short exercise time;

Wednesday is the day for grocery shopping, doctor's appointments and other errands. Next plan time for yourself. Once everyone is acquainted and satisfied with the routine, you can plan for relief help. Visitors will soon learn when best to call.

Note: You might prepare copies of the weekly schedule for the one you care for, family members and the friends who visit. Add a little drawing and print "We have time for a visit every day. Please stop by."

Help with Personal Care

As you prepare to help your loved one, be sure to wash your hands. Next try to group activities together so you do not walk empty-handed from place to place.

The Bath

You know how to help with a bath, but here are a few suggestions and time-saving tips for giving a bath to someone lying in bed or sitting in a chair:

- Gather everything you will need before you start. Keep the bath area warm and draft-free.

- Ask about elimination. If an enema is needed, the person can evacuate with little straining while sitting on the bathroom commode or on a bedside commode chair.

- The bath water should be very warm, or as warm as is still comfortable on your elbow.

- Use a small amount of mild soap, rinse well, and dry. You are removing perspiration, primarily, and stimulating circulation.

- Give your loved one a sponge instead of a wash cloth if he uses one hand to assist with the bath. It is easier to squeeze water out of a sponge.

- Use baby powder, not corn starch, following the bath. The mineral oil in baby powder does not promote yeast growth (especially for a person whose illness makes them susceptible to yeast spores).

- If his or her feet appear dry and "scaly" between baths, soak in a basin of warm, soapy water. Rinse, dry thoroughly and apply a moisturizer. Try the emulsion (with Crisco) as described under "Tips to Protect the Skin" on page 16.

- If a loved one is obese, use a hand-held hair dryer, set on LOW, and dry in the folds or under the breasts. Be careful that the skin doesn't get too hot.

One quick and easy method for giving a bed bath:

- Fill a large basin with very warm water and add one to two ounces of lanolin-based liquid soap. Wet three (3) wash cloths and one (1) bath towel. Wring out and place in a large plastic bag.

- Use one washcloth for face, neck, arms and hands. Dry with a soft bath towel.

- Place the wet bath towel over the front of the body and massage gently. Dry well.

- Use the second wash cloth to cleanse the perineal and groin area. Dry gently and thoroughly.

- Turn the person on his side. Use the third wash cloth to wash the back and buttocks. Dry thoroughly.

- Select one of the wash cloths to wash the legs and feet. Dry well, especially between the toes.

Note: You may substitute a hand towel for the wash cloth to wash the back and buttocks. Also a lanolin-based soap does not need to be removed. If another type of soap is used, fill a basin with warm water and rinse all soap off before drying.

Washing Hair While in Bed

Washing a loved one's hair when they are lying in bed requires ingenuity. Here is an easy method:

Lower the head of the bed as flat as can be tolerated. Slip a pillow under the shoulders so the neck rests comfortably. Place a large plastic trash bag on the bed, over the pillow and down under the shoulders. Cover the plastic bag with a small towel for comfort. Slip a plastic vegetable bin, with a half circle cut out of one side, under the head and neck. Pad the rim of the half circle with a small hand towel. Shampoo, rinse and let water drain into the bin.

You may substitute a large trash bag for the vegetable bin. Move the person at an angle on the bed so the water will drain into a large wastebasket on the floor. Roll a large bath towel and curve the roll around his head, then cover the area under the head and over the rolled towel with a trash bag. Let the end of the bag drape over the side of the bed and rest in a wastebasket.

Note: Use a hair conditioner to help prevent tangles and rinse well. Comb the hair gently with a large-toothed plastic comb. You may find products in the drugstore and supermarket for cleansing the hair without soap or water.

Help with a Tub Bath

It is safer to sit in an arm chair by the bathroom sink for a sponge bath than to climb into a tub. However, when the person prefers to get in the tub, find a bath seat with rubber grippers or place a length of foam "egg crate" in the bottom of the tub. If the hips remain higher than the feet, it is easier to exit from the tub. An inexpensive hand-held shower head makes showering easy and a grab bar that is attached to the wall or the front of the tub provides safety.

- Do not add more hot water as the water cools. Short baths prevent fatigue. Ask your patient if he feels light-headed. Let the water out, dry the arms and upper body and wrap a towel around his hips. Offer a steadying hand as he steps out of the tub. You may hold around the waist (stand on the weaker side) as he exits the tub if he seems unsteady. The person may choose to sit on the side of the tub and swing one leg over at a time. Dry the rest of his body.

- You may wrap your loved one in a full-length terry robe as he or she steps out of the tub. It is warm, will absorb water and you only need dry under breasts, in the groin area, and the feet.

- Check body alignment when the person returns to bed. Stand at the foot of the bed and check that the body is not twisted, paralyzed limbs are being supported, and toes are not bound by the top covers. Poor body alignment soon causes discomfort.

- Cut the crown out of a plastic shower cap for a person who cannot tilt his head back far enough to keep soap out of his eyes and ears as the hair is washed. Place the cap on the head as usual and let the edges drop down.

- Before showering, cover any area of skin that must remain dry (IV site, dressing etc.) with a disposable diaper, panty shield or a small zip lock bag. The plastic side of the pad should be away from the skin. Tape all edges carefully so the area will remain dry while bathing.

Tips to Protect the Skin

- To prevent dry, calloused skin, especially on the feet, use a skin moisturizer or cream:
  - An inexpensive cream is made by using a solid vegetable shortening such as Crisco. Put a small amount of the shortening in the palm of your hand, add a few drops of warm water and mix until it forms a creamy emulsion.

When rubbed in the skin, it does not leave a greasy coating.

— Two products, Bag Balm and Corona cream, found in farm product stores and many drugstores, have excellent healing qualities for irritated skin. One store owner commented that he now sells more of these products for diaper rash than for healing cows' teats.

- To prevent skin irritations caused by wearing various types of splints or braces use well-worn socks for padding.
  — For a hand splint, cut the sock's toe off and make a hole in the heel. Slip the thumb through the hole in the heel and slip the fingers through the cut-off toe. Apply the splint.
  — To prevent leg brace irritations, cut one leg from an old panty hose and remove the foot. Pull the hose over the calf or thigh to hold the padding in place. Slip a piece of fake fur, quilted batting, or spongy blanket material inside the hose where a brace rubs the skin. Apply the splint or leg brace.
  — To prevent bruises, chafed elbows or reddened skin on the forearms, remove the toe from a soft athletic or other type sock. Slip the sock over the arm so that the heel of the sock covers the elbow.

- To remove sticky substances from the skin:
  — Remove tape from the skin by saturating a cotton ball with alcohol and rubbing gently.
  — Remove any dried bowel movement from the skin by placing a small amount of hand or baby lotion on a soft cloth and rubbing gently.

Bedmaking Made Easy

How many beds have you made during your lifetime? More than you want to remember? Check the number of times that you move from one side of the bed to the other. Here are some labor-saving tips:

- **Save time and extra steps.**
  Place the pillows and all linens on one side of the bed.
  Start by slipping the fitted bottom sheet on each end of the mattress; place the top sheet over it. You may knot the bottom corner of the top sheet or tuck the sheet under the mattress. You have one-half of the linens in place. Move the rest of each sheets to the middle of the bed. Put pillow cases on all of the pillows and set aside.
  Walk to the other side of the bed. Slip the other two corners of the bottom sheet over the mattress. Tuck or tie the bottom of the top sheet. Place the pillows in place. Finally, add the spread or comforter.

- **Use padding for comfort and mattress protection.**
  People arrive home from the hospital with an "egg crate" foam pad. You did bring it, didn't you? It has been purchased by the patient, as are the basins, bed pan and other items in the admission kit. This popular, inexpensive mattress pad may be found in linen departments, medical supply stores and catalogues. The egg crate design stimulates circulation, relieves pressure from bony prominences and adds comfort. Cover the pad with a fitted bottom sheet (only) for best results. You may add a large disposable pad if dribbling is a problem or add a folded sheet for lifting. The ridged foam pad is washable. Use a small amount of soap, rinse, and spin on the gentle cycle. Dry in the dryer on a cool cycle for a few minutes. If the elevated ridges flatten from pressure, hold a hair dryer over the area for a few minutes and the foam peaks will puff up again.

  Note: To make a lift or draw sheet, fold a large, flat sheet once or twice and placed under the person from shoulders to below the hips. To lift, one person stands on each side, grasps the lift sheet and pulls steadily against each other. The bedfast person's body will be elevated off the mattress just high enough to be easily moved up in bed. Changing the draw sheet and pillow case may be all that is needed to freshen the bed at the end of the day.

- Sheets need to be smooth and dry. A new, inexpensive product keeps bottom sheets wrinkle free. It is a strip of wide elastic with a clamp or fastener on each end. Attached at an angle across the corners of the bottom sheet under the mattress, it keeps the sheet smooth and tight. You can easily make four sheet clips if you are a seamstress.

- When a loved one has night sweats or perspires frequently, a polyester and cotton sheet may become uncomfortable and irritate or "sting" the skin. Substitute soft cotton sheets, thin cotton blankets or old, soft muslin sheets.

- Waterbeds offer a comfortable, more pressure-free bed, but unless surrounded by a firm, formed side shell, a loved one may have some difficulty getting out of bed. Place a quilted mattress pad over a plastic waterbed and tuck the bottom sheet far under the mattress.

  Note: When my son was paralyzed and waiting for admission to a rehab center, we placed an inexpensive air mattress over the cushions on our long living room couch. The mattress was inflated until his hips did not touch the cushions below. The mattress was covered with a quilted pad and sheet (which were pinned and tucked under the mattress.) Three pillows were added at one end. A light weight comforter became the top cover. When he grew tired of sitting in his wheelchair, the makeshift bed permitted him to be in the midst of our family's activities.

- Caregivers often look for inexpensive substitutes for the

large disposable pads needed when a person is incontinent (or might dribble urine when they cough.) To keep the mattress or chair seat dry, try an inexpensive, commonly-used product. Purchase a long, flannel-backed plastic table cloth and place crosswise over the bed, leaving the flannel side exposed. Tuck the ends under the sides of the mattress, or if not long enough, sew material (strips of old sheets, etc.) on each end. Adjust the size to fit a chair seat. Wash in cool water on the gentle cycle and dry for a few minutes in the dryer. Finish by air-drying.

A second substitute (and my favorite) is the double or single-sided, waterproof, flannel pads which are used on a baby's beds. They make excellent pads, since the double-sided flannel (with waterproof material in the center) clings to the bed's bottom sheet. Look for the material by the yard in fabric stores. Pink the edges. These pads wash well and last for many months.

- Top covers should be lightweight and fit loosely over the toes. Toes tend to drop down when lying in bed, especially if covers are tucked in, and the danger increases that the inactive muscles which attach to the heel, may shorten. Ignored, a loved one may have difficulty walking again and may require prolonged physical therapy to recover. To prevent foot drop:
  — Tie a loose knot in each bottom corner of the top bed sheet so it will fit loosely. Do not tuck under the mattress.

    Place well-filled pillows or a padded board against the soles of the feet. Several times a day (if leg is not injured) place your open palms against the bottom of each foot and push the toes forward, gently and steadily, several times. This exercise tightens the thigh and calf muscles normally used in walking. The doctor may order high top walking shoes to be worn for several hours each day. Lined, firm-soled house slippers will also offer support and protect from foot drop.

— A comforter makes an excellent light weight top cover. It offers as much warmth as a quilt or blanket, but with less weight. A comforter is easily made, even by someone who does not sew. A disabled loved one might enjoy making one.

Directions:

Use two sheets, new or used, and add a layer of batting between them. Polyester batting is available in a roll and may be cut in any length. To cover a double bed, use the larger queen-size sheets. Using 2-inch quilting pins, pin through the three layers every 10-12 inches. Alternate on the next row. Thread a large needle with two strands of yarn and take a short stitch where each pin is located. Knot the yarn with a double square knot to anchor the layers together. The outside edges may be overcast together or closed by folding and ironing "Stitch Witchery" between them. Colorful fabric (45"x72") makes equally comfortable lap robes. These comforters wash well and remain fluffy.

• Small pillows have many uses. They provide support under a shoulder, elbow, neck, in the small of the back, under the edge of a hip, between the knees, or under an ankle. To make several small pillows, try this quick method:

Purchase an inexpensive polyester-filled bed pillow. Cut the cover completely around the center, pull some of the batting from the opened area, and pin the opened ends together. You now have two smaller pillows that are fluffy and full or soft and thin depending on the amount of batting removed. Stitch the raw edges together or iron with "Stitch Witchery." You may need several pillows of various sizes. Take your old pillowcases, cut in two equal lengths crosswise and close one end. You have pillowcases that fit the small pillows.

Correct Body Positioning

Young and healthy people may fall asleep in awkward positions, awaken, stretch and walk away. However, a body with weakened or paralyzed muscles lacks the ability to lift and reposition itself.

You should observe a loved one, then help position his body in a good, straight alignment when he sits or lies in bed. Good body alignment prevents joint deformities, muscle aches and spasms, headaches, and skin breakdown. The body's weight should be evenly distributed over as much of the bed or chair surface as possible. Points to remember:

- Encourage a disabled loved one to move his body as much as he is able until he finds a comfortable position. Add pillows to hold the position.

- The spine should remain straight when sitting or lying down.

  Support the small of the back. Paralyzed arms and legs are heavy and seem to be a "dead weight." They require special support:

  — When sitting in a chair or in bed, place a pillow under the the person's elbow to remove the pull on the shoulder joint.

  — Rest the hand on the paralyzed side on a pillow. Elevating the hand prevents swelling.

  — While lying on his back, place one pillow folded lengthwise under the outer thigh of a paralyzed leg. A second pillow may be placed under the calf or a small pillow under the ankle to keep pressure off the heel. Remember to push gently on the toes.

  — When the person is sitting in bed, elevate the bed at the knees to prevent him from sliding down. Ask the doctor if it is safe to place a pillow under the knees when lying in a regular bed.

— Check to determine that the person is breathing easily and does not have a heavy, paralyzed arm lying across the chest.

- Stand at the foot of the bed or in front of your patient's chair. Observe the body's position and ask the patient if he is comfortable or feels "strained." Muscles will tighten to prevent the body from leaning to one side, tire, and begin to ache. As he sits in a chair, position the hips against the back of the chair. The body's weight should be supported on the upper thighs and buttocks. The back of the knees should not press against the edge of the chair seat. Both feet should be placed flat on the floor, on a footrest or on telephone books if the person is short. The patient who spends several hours in a chair should move or rock from side to side frequently (about every 30-45 minutes) to improve circulation.

When You Move a Loved One

Caregiver's injuries are often due to lifting mistakes. Learn the correct way to help your loved one sit up in bed, to lift him up in bed alone or with someone's help, to help him move safely from bed to chair and to help him back into bed. Books on basic care are available in the library and bookstores. One book with concise instructions and excellent illustrations is titled *Caring for the Sick: Nursing the Ill, the Disabled, Children and the Elderly* by Ellen Lagala. If you cannot find the book you need, ask the librarian for a library to library transfer, which is a free service.

Other tips for moving a weak, disabled person include:

- Tell your loved one what you are going to do. Explain how he can help and reassure him you will support and not drop him.

- Before turning your patient on his side, place a chair back

against the bed for a handhold support and to prevent his
rolling out of bed.

- Stay close to your work. Stand close, put your arm firmly
  around the person for support when he needs it. Place the
  chair or wheelchair (with wheels locked) sideways against
  the bed before transferring him into it.

- Lift by holding the joints, such as an elbow, wrist, knee
  or ankle, rather than the soft tissue. If a bruise develops,
  consider where you have been holding when you lift. Reach
  completely under a shoulder or under a hip before lifting
  someone sideways toward you. Don't pull on an arm or leg
  as you try to move his body.

- Encourage the person to move as much as he is able. He
  may move a paralyzed arm by grasping it with the other
  strong hand or his leg by slipping a strong foot under a
  paralyzed ankle and lifting. The more he is able to help
  himself, the less helpless he will feel.

- Remind your loved one to sit quietly for a few minutes
  when first sitting up after lying in bed. This time permits the
  blood pressure to adjust and prevents dizziness or a possible
  fall when he transfers to a chair or starts to walk.

How to Give a Relaxing Back Rub

A good back rub, given with the heels of your hands in strong, even
strokes, will relax muscles, calm nerves, leave one with a sense of
well being and help induce sleep. Muscles grow tired after one sits in a
chair or lies in bed for hours. Massage relaxes them. Try the following
technique:

- Raise the head of the hospital bed slightly and stand at an
  angle facing the head of the bed. Or sit on the side of a low,
  double bed. Turn the person on the side away from you. Put
  a cream, lotion or rubbing alcohol (feels cool, tends to dry

and toughen the skin) in the palms of your hands. Check for any reddened areas, bruises or breaks in the skin.

- Starting at the waist, use the heels of both hands and maintain a firm, even pressure as you stroke upward toward the back of the neck. Then circle over the shoulder blades and back down over the heavy muscles that lie along each side of the spine. Keep a firm, even pressure under the heel of the hand. Continue to circle downward and out over the hip bones. Unless the area is reddened, massage deeply. Repeat with variations: massage the back of the neck and out along the top of the shoulders, make circles over the shoulder blades and move down to the waist. Massage in circles in the small of the back. Look for breaks in the skin or whitened areas over bony prominences, and do not massage these areas.

Note: Force is not needed - do not push your patient out of bed. Keep lotion or alcohol on your hands so they will not pull or "drag" on the skin. Use even, smooth strokes to reach the underlying muscles but do not cause discomfort. Do not use your fingertips. Be very gentle if you massage any reddened areas.

All family members, can learn to give a beneficial back rub. Offer to let them practice on a tired caregiver. When sleep eludes a disabled loved one, try a back rub, soft music and kind words to help them fall asleep.

A Relaxation Technique

A disability may confine one to a chair, bed or house for hours or days at a time. The disabled individual's choice of activities is limited, life grows boring, muscles ache, food loses its appeal and by bedtime he cannot relax. When you have given a back rub, brought warm milk and helped make him comfortable, and he is still awake; try a simple, effective relaxation technique:

Turn the sound of instrumental music just loud enough to close out other sounds. Be sure the person is as comfortable as possible, smooth sheets, fluff pillows (change a damp pillow case) and loosen the top covers. Ask him to close his eyes and listen to your voice. Start by asking your loved one to place himself in a place which he has enjoyed. He may remember floating in a boat, lying on the grass under an old elm tree or wherever he found comfort and peace.

You begin by explaining how relaxed he will feel; then what he is feeling; and finally what has been accomplished. Start by explaining how calm and relaxed he will become. Ask him to listen to the quiet music and let it fill the mind. Quietly tell the person that his body is growing lighter, almost weightless, as though he is floating. Reinforce the warm, unencumbered and free feeling by slowly repeating the instructions. Observe his body and note if it is relaxing. You may continue to describe tense areas that are relaxing. His mind will become quieted, freed from thoughts and cares as the music washes over him. Speak slowly with pauses which allow time for the body to respond to your suggestions.

Finally, explain that he is letting go, relaxing completely and has become sleepy. If not actually asleep, he will have calmed his mind of anxieties and will more easily fall asleep. Once your loved one understands how the mind helps the body relax, he will feel a greater measure of control as he helps himself relax and rest.

Note: Use your own words, do not discuss or offer too many details. Speak softly, slowly and make the words easily understood. Try to have a rhythm or cadence to the words. Do not hurry.

Don't feel uncomfortable when you try a relaxation technique. I assured my teen-age granddaughter that I could help her get to sleep. I started at the top of her head and explained that each part of her body was relaxing, and she was asleep before I reached her toes. She would ask me to repeat the technique until I reminded her that she could help herself.

I attended a nursing conference on relaxation where the participants enjoyed a relaxation scenario. All but two of the nurses fell asleep. Everyone felt relaxed and invigorated and were surprised that the technique was so effective.

Controlling Acute or Chronic Pain

Many people who live with a disabling condition or a chronic illness escape an unwanted companion - chronic pain. Those who do not understand pain, don't realize it makes its victim anxious and sleepless. Unrelieved, the pain becomes a controller, shutting its victim into a self-centered world of consuming misery. Pain is a symptom, a protector, that informs us when our body is not functioning properly.

A person's reaction to mild pain is usually different than it is to severe pain. Mild pain makes one restless, short-tempered or slightly depressed. He may lie quietly or may become more talkative.

With moderate to severe pain the person may moan, cry or become angry. He may react by describing each sharp pain or may insist on privacy. Individually, the victim reacts to pain as he has reacted to other crises in his life.

Endorphins, the body's own pain relievers, play a role in both inhibiting painful stimuli and actually controlling pain. Researchers suspect that the amount of pain we feel is based on our endorphin level - the higher the level, the less pain. Continuing pain may deplete our endorphin level. The level may be influenced (lowered) when a person is severely depressed. Since chronic pain tends to make the sufferer feel depressed, a vicious cycle may be created.

Your loved one's pain may be chronic, intermittent or it may grow progressively more severe. Pain, untreated, becomes nerve-racking. Before you call the doctor you should:

- Ask him to pinpoint the exact location of the pain. Deep aching pain may be harder to pinpoint.

- Ask for a description of the pain - throbbing, burning, cutting, aching, shooting, cramping, gnawing, boring, squeezing, etc.

> Superficial pain is often described as sharp or tingling, while deep, internal pain is a dull, constant ache.

- Ask him to rate the intensity of the pain, how severe it feels, on a scale of one to five. Five is very severe or almost unbearable.

- Ask other questions: Has he felt nauseated? Had a headache or felt dizzy? Been constipated or had diarrhea?

> **Note:** The above answers are your loved one's and your observations are equally important. Does he hold himself very still or is he continuously moving around? Is he frowning with the mouth held tightly and the corners pulled down? Does he have a "pinched" anxious look? Has his pulse rate and respirations increased?

The person in pain may be unable to talk to you, due to confusion, aphasia or semi-consciousness. You must watch his expressions and check his movements very carefully. He may fall asleep from exhaustion and still be experiencing pain.

When you call the doctor make an accurate and concise report, without injecting many of your own opinions. The doctor may ask if pain has affected his appetite or his ability to get a good night's sleep. The doctor may wish to see him in person.

Treating the Pain

The doctor will balance the strength of the medication with the severity of the pain. Medications should bring relief in 20-40 minutes and if adequate, will keep the person free from pain for about 3-1/2 to 4 hours. Notify the doctor if the person is not relieved and continues to have moderate pain; or if he becomes uncomfortable again in two to three hours. The medication has not been adequate for the amount and intensity of his pain, and the doctor needs to be informed so that a more effective medication (or combination of medicines) may be ordered.

Please remember: A pain medication is "used up" by the pain that is present, and will not cause an addiction. It is only when the person has little or no pain, but continues to take heavy narcotics (as with drug abusers) that an addiction will develop. An emotional dependence is different from a physical dependence.

Actions that Allow Needless Pain:

- The person decides to suffer pain without relief. His nerves become ragged, he feels exhausted and more depressed. But still he refuses to take a medication in the mistaken belief that he will become an addict. His ignorance is harming him.

- The caregiver adheres strictly to the four-hour order, despite the patient's obvious misery, because of her fear of addiction. Pain is a subjective experience and only the victim feels his pain. If the caregiver suspects that the person has magnified his complaints out of fear, she should check his pulse and blood pressure, then inform the doctor. The doctor is the pain control expert and understands that emotional pain is real and can become intertwined with physical pain.

  Note: Do not arbitrarily lengthen the time between doses of medicine without speaking with the doctor. When pain becomes mild or intermittent, the doctor may change the drug to a mild pain reliever.

A Word of Caution:

Medications are frequently given in combination, allowing a smaller dose of narcotic to be accentuated or prolonged by another non-narcotic medication. Always fill the prescriptions that the doctor has ordered. To save money, ask if a generic version is available. Do not mix over-the-counter pain relievers, one borrowed from a friend, or an old medication from a dental appointment with the new prescription medicines for pain.

Techniques To Help an Uncomfortable Loved One Relax

Try distraction. Through experience, you have learned how to distract others by changing the subject or interesting a child in another activity. Distraction provides a kind of "sensory shield" if a loved one has mild or chronic pain. It prevents a full awareness of pain and consequently, increases his tolerance of it. Relief lasts only as long as he is distracted. Once ended, he may feel tired and is once again aware of the continuing pain. Try one of the following distraction techniques if he is restless and uncomfortable while waiting for the pain medication to take effect.

- Ask your loved one to recall an exciting event, family gathering or movie he or she enjoyed. You might start by asking, "Do you remember ..."

- Suggest that he use earphones and turn the radio or tape player louder when the pain is stronger and lower when the pain diminishes. Also suggest that he tap his fingers or nod his head to the music. This kind of distraction blocks out other sounds so one can concentrate on the words. (Teenagers seem to have perfected this technique.)

- Deep breathing is both distracting and relaxing. Ask the person to close his eyes, visualize a lovely, quiet place and describe it.

  Note: These may seem to be simple techniques. Once practiced with relaxing results, your loved one will feel more in control. With fewer anxious moments, the body is better able to mobilize its own defenses against pain. The person might require less medication.

Technique for Head-to-Toe Relaxation

Prepare your loved one by smoothing and tightening the linens, handing him a very warm, wet washcloth to wipe his face and hands and helping him get comfortable.

This technique, while similar to others, has the person concentrating on relaxing each area of the body. Explain that his muscles have grown tired and need to relax. He deserves to rest and renew his body. Ask the person to take a deep breath, exhale completely and repeat several more slow, deep breaths. Starting at the head, explain that the eyes are shut with the lids relaxed, the jaw muscles loosen and relax and the muscles around the mouth soften and relax. The neck has grown tired of supporting the head and relaxes so the head may sink into the pillow.

Speak slowly and gently as you pause often for him to let his body respond to your words. Describe how first the shoulders, then arms and hands are relaxing and become heavier. Continue these instructions for the back, legs, feet and toes. Watch the body relax as his mind understands your words. If an area remains tense, such as the legs remain drawn up, explain further. Reinforce that the body is now relaxed, is warm and comfortable and the person feels as though they are lying on a soft featherbed. Take your time to help relax the body. This is a technique that once he experiences it, the person may be able to do for himself.

Two Home Remedies for Relief of Minor Pain

- **Cold packs.**

  Cold offers quicker and longer-lasting relief in many instances than the customary use of hot packs. Try one for a headache, sore throat, joint pain from immobility, muscle spasms or chronic pain. Wrap an ice bag a frozen, wet washcloth or a small bag of frozen vegetables with a small towel or other cloth.

- **Apply a menthol ointment.**

  No one is sure how it relieves pain; whether it is the aspirin-like ingredient found in most of them, the sensation produced that overrides the pain, or a placebo effect. It does offer relief. It helps relieve joint pain and it might be rubbed on the back of the neck or forehead for a tension headache. People in the Far East will rub some on the abdomen to relieve gas pains. The menthol produces a warm sensation (sometimes coolness) that may last for hours.

Chapter Four

WHEN TIME MUST BE SPENT IN BED

Our bodies were created to be active, and when they are not, for whatever reason, we may develop problems. The changes or complications which may result from inactivity are described in this chapter. The alert caregiver strives to prevent complications through early treatment.

A person who is disabled, whether from a stroke, spinal cord injury, acute arthritic episode, advanced cancer, complications from AIDS or the weakness from advanced age, may require bed rest for varying periods of time. Our body was not designed to remain horizontal or to have restricted motion for a long time. Remaining in bed becomes a scenario for complications - unless action is taken.

The body needs to move as much as it is able. Your loved one needs to walk, with or without help, sit in a wheelchair or bedside chair, or sit on the side of the bed. If he or she is so weak that they need continuous bed rest, raise and lower the head of the bed several times during the day.

The following changes and complications can be prevented or minimized despite spending most of each day in bed:

- The pulse rate may drop. If an inactive person sits up quickly, he may feel weak, faint or dizzy, and the skin may be cold and clammy. Give your patient a few minutes for the circulation to adjust to an upright position.

- Breathing tends to become shallower. There is a danger that fluids may tend to collect in the lungs with the decreased chest movements.

- The bladder may become distended and may allow urine to leak. Urine output increases as does the loss of calcium from the body.

- Muscles start to weaken, especially those used for standing and walking.

- The urge to have a bowel movement grows weaker, so the lower bowel contents gradually becomes dryer and firmer. The person may waste energy straining to empty the lower bowel and may develop painful hemorrhoids.

- Circulation becomes poorer when he or she is bedfast, so the person should exercise in bed to prevent any small blood clots from forming.

- The danger of forming pressure (bed) sores increases.

- The other internal body systems are also affected: insulin production may drop, hormones tend to stop working properly, body fluids tend to shift and some neurological changes may take place.

- Perhaps of greater importance, the person restricted to bed feels helpless and dependent. He soon feels isolated, tends to become introspective and will focus more and more on his illness.

The following simple procedures will help prevent these complications:

Lung complications

Our lungs act as a two-way bellows when we walk, but when we lie in bed, the lungs tend to compress slightly. After a few weeks, the oxygen intake may decrease by as much as one-fourth. Any pooled secretions will tend to thicken, increasing the danger of pneumonia.

You can prevent lung complications by elevating the head of a hospital-type bed about one-third (30-45 degree angle) for short periods several times a day. In a regular bed, place two pillows in an inverted V, and add a third or even a fourth pillow crosswise across the V. If the person is strong enough, help him sit on the side of the bed. Encourage, coax and plead with him to take slow, deep breaths throughout the day.

Deep breathing is best done by inhaling slowly through the nose, then exhaling slowly with the mouth slightly opened and the lips pursed to form a small 0. Another effective method, especially for someone with a chronic lung condition, is to push or pull the abdomen out when inhaling, (which seems the opposite of normal breathing,) and let it relax as they exhale.

Note: One person may be able to breathe more deeply than another but the effort should be made. If you hear changes, such as repeated rattling or wheezing with each breath, take his vital signs (temperature, pulse and respirations) and report the information to the doctor (or hospice nurse).

Blood Circulation Complications

As the heart pumps blood throughout the body, muscle movement, especially leg muscles, helps the blood return to the heart. Lying quietly in bed for many hours permits the blood to start pooling in the legs and other areas.

The best protection against complications is to get out of bed. If the person is unable to do so, moving the toes and heels up and down, turning and repositioning will help improve circulation. Remove constricting clothing, elevate the patient's legs while sitting and change positions frequently. The doctor may order elasticized stockings for someone who is bedfast. The stockings should be rolled on, kept free of wrinkles or twisting and changed daily.

Skin and Underlying Tissue Complications

The skin frequently suffers when time is spent in bed. Skin may chafe or be "burned" when a bottom sheet is accidentally jerked from under the person. Burns occur most often on the buttocks, heel, shoulder, elbow or even the ear - areas which have the body's weight on them in bed. The burn is painful, forms a scar and takes time to heal.

Each caregiver may believe that someone else has turned the bedfast loved one, who remained in the same position for five or six hours. Despite your best efforts, if the oversight or neglect is repeated, it will allow a thin, aged skin and the tissue under it, to break down. The skin will turn red, and if the pressure is not relieved, will turn white. Finally, the injured skin and tissue breaks down and fluid weeps from the area. A pressure ulcer "bedsore" develops due to the compression of small blood vessels. The area has been deprived of both oxygen and nutrients. The injured area must be treated gently and will require weeks or months of consistent treatment to heal. Many doctors have a favorite treatment regimen that they prescribe.

A reddened, "scalded" area may appear when perspiration remains under pendulous breasts, urine is not washed from groins or a bowel movement (especially liquid BM) remains on the buttocks for some time. The skin barrier against bacteria and future infection is broken. The damaged skin must be protected and treated quickly.

You can prevent skin breakdown. Pull a sheet slowly and steadily from beneath a bedfast loved one. Ask someone to help lift and turn him, using a folded full-size sheet for a draw sheet. Check frequently for perspiration and wrinkled or wet sheets. Gently wash the skin, rinse well, pat dry and powder. Put lotion on elbows, knees and feet.

To help prevent bedsores, cover the mattress with an "egg crate," synthetic sheep skin, air mattress or alternating pressure pad. Protect the skin from a plastic cover. Help the person turn from side to side every few hours. Check the skin when the person turns and if reddened, gently massage the area. If a whitened area is noted, turn immediately but DO NOT massage the area. Check in a short while to see if the skin has regained a pink color.

Note: The staff of one large nursing home was proud that the only pressure sores found on patients in their center were those seen on admission or following a hospital stay. The staff would immediately begin treatment, and in time the sore was healed. Every patient who spent time in bed had a turning schedule, was kept dry and clean. Any reddened skin area was treated as ordered by the doctor. Mattresses were covered by "egg crates" and patients were given adequate fluids, juices and food supplements. The nursing home staff had no secrets, just careful observation and dependable routine care.

If the skin is broken, for whatever reason, contact the doctor and treat exactly as ordered. Healing requires time and effort, but the denuded skin area will heal (starting from the bottom of the crater or sore) with consistent daily care.

Elimination Complications

Inactivity and bed rest create problems for the body's elimination system. The distended bladder may not empty completely and the residual urine provides an opportunity for bacteria to grow. The sluggish bowel may cause loss of appetite, nausea and bloating. Laxatives, enemas and in rare cases, manual removal, may be required to evacuate the lower bowel. Tips for prevention or treatment include:

- Establish a routine for voiding. Help your patient sit up, if possible, and press over the bladder area to help emptying. Serve hot fluids as well as cold. Dilute cranberry juice with water and serve 3-4 ounces daily.

- Review your loved one's medications (including over-the-counter) with the pharmacist for any that are prone to cause constipation. List any laxatives used repeatedly over a period of time. If you find one which may cause elimination problems, ask the doctor if it can be changed or reduced.

- Provide adequate liquids daily. These include tea, coffee, juices, Jello, soup, skimmed milk, supplements such as Ensure and water. Omit tomato or V8 juice unless listed as low sodium.

- Serve fruit daily and include dried fruits (raisins, prunes, etc.) as well as fresh or canned. Add whole grain cereals and bread for bulk, but exclude plain bran for a bedfast person.

General Problems with Elimination

A person often creates problems in an effort to maintain good elimination. "Normal" elimination varies from voiding every two to three hours and having a bowel movement daily, to double those times. If urine is held for eight hours before voiding, the waste products start to break down. When the lower bowel is not emptied for several days, the body has time to reabsorb extra water from the bowel contents, making the stool firmer. It is the conditions outside the norm, frequent and uncomfortable voidings, diarrhea and severe constipation that become problems.

Recognizing Symptoms of Problems

Cystitis occurs when the bladder is irritated or infected. Early symptoms include an urgent need to void quickly and often (without drinking extra fluids) and may be accompanied by burning and cramping. The person should "flush the bladder" by drinking extra water, unless liquids are limited, and might include 3-4 ounces of cranberry juice two or three times daily. A prescribed medicine for cystitis will stop the miserable symptoms and end a bladder infection. Check if the temperature is elevated.

Diarrhea occurs when the bowel contents move quickly through the colon and three or more watery stools are experienced over a 24-hour period. The body will dehydrate, and with babies and the fragile elderly, it can soon become a medical emergency. The discomfort and weakness makes one feel miserable enough to lose interest in food or replacement fluids. Nausea and vomiting will compound the problem. Contact the doctor if diarrhea continues over 24-hours.

Symptoms of Constipation

If a person who usually has a bowel movement daily has no BM for two or three days, elimination may be uncomfortable and exhausting. Without relief, the abdomen distends with a gas buildup, cramping begins and brings on a loss of appetite. A more serious condition develops with prolonged constipation. The dry, hardened stool cannot be expelled without strenuous, repeated straining and may need to be broken up (with a gloved finger) before the person can expel it.

Factors that influence elimination are well known. The disabled person who sits in a chair or lies in bed most of the day, the elderly person who does not exercise and has weakened abdominal muscles, and the person who prefers soft, bland foods and forgets to drink enough fluids may all have problems with chronic constipation. Constant emotional stress may trigger episodes of diarrhea.

In an effort to have a normal elimination, people tend to overuse laxatives and other over-the-counter drugs. Seniors frequently decide that a "good cleaning out" is as valuable as the "spring tonic" taken years ago.

Correcting Constipation

You should be familiar with your loved one's normal evacuation routine and if an extra day or two passes without a BM, try the following:

- Choose a time about one-half hour after a hot meal. The reflexes which push bowel contents toward the rectum are more active after eating hot food.

- Ask the person to place both hands across the lower abdomen (if able to do so) lean forward and compress the abdomen against the thighs.

- To help stimulate the reflex for elimination, suggest that they gently massage the anal sphincter, pinch the inner thigh or pull on the pubic hair.

- If none of these tips work, let them relax and try again in an hour or two.

You should ask your loved one each day if he has had a BM. If two or three days go by without results, discuss the problem with the doctor. A laxative may be ordered which will act on the large intestine to increase the speed at which the contents pass through the bowel, to increase its bulk and/or its water contents.

Types of Laxatives

- **Bulk-forming**
  A relatively slow-acting laxative which is less likely to interfere with normal bowel action. The person should drink a full glass of water or juice with it and wait two hours before taking other medicines. It is usually taken in the morning. Examples: Metamucil, Modane Bulk.

- **Lubricant**
  A stool softener may be ordered when a hard stool causes pain (as with hemorrhoids). It is often recommended for an elderly or debilitated person, and for the relief of a fecal impaction. A stool softener may interfere to some degree with the absorption of the fat-soluble vitamins A, D, E and K. It is to be taken at bedtime in fruit juice or a carbonated

drink. Do not give these over a week unless prescribed by the doctor. Example: mineral oil.

- **Saline Laxative**
  It acts to pull water back into the intestine and speed movement through the colon. You should shake the suspension well and insist that the person drink plenty of water. Wait two hours before giving medicines. Do not give over a period of time without approval from the doctor. Example: Milk of Magnesia.

- **Emollient**
  A laxative which allows oil and water to mix with bowel contents to promote the formation of a soft, formed stool. It helps relieve chronic constipation and prevents straining. Do not give with mineral oil or other oil products. It should be taken at bedtime and not with other medicines. Examples: Colace, Peri-colace, Doxidan.

- **Stimulating**
  This quick acting laxative may be ordered when other treatments have failed. The person may experience abdominal cramps and diarrhea. It is to be taken at bedtime with a snack and usually only for a short period of time. If taken with a medicine for high blood pressure (such as a diuretic) it may lower the potassium level. Examples: Senokot, Dr. Caldwell's Senna Laxative, Black Draught.

An Example of an Effective Plan:

A man in his nineties who resided in a nursing home followed a simple routine that was effective for him. He took a small dose of Milk of Magnesia with his evening meal and Peri-colace (or a generic substitute) at bedtime. Prior to his shower every three days, he was helped to the commode chair and given time for a BM. If he could not evacuate, an enema was given the next morning but was seldom necessary. He also took a multivitamin/mineral supplement daily.

Note: When you contact the doctor because your loved one has become constipated or has had watery stools for two days (a 24-hour period for children or elderly):

— Describe any pain or discomfort, bowel movements that have changes in color (black, chalk colored, etc.) or other problems, such as hemorrhoids.

— Ask which laxative he or she recommends. Ask if there are any that your loved one should not be given.

— After a bout of diarrhea, ask what should be taken as replacement for fluid and mineral losses.

Bowel Impaction

Suspect a bowel impaction when a person (especially one who spends most of his day in a wheelchair or bed) has the following symptoms:

— Has not had a bowel movement for four or five days.
— Has an abdomen that is noticeably distended.
— Has loss of appetite and feels miserable.
— May pass a small amount of watery stool. A watery stool may build up behind the hard, obstructing stool and will leak around it.

If you suspect an impaction, you should:

— Slip on a clean plastic or rubber glove and spread a lubricant, such as K-Y Jelly (I use baby oil) over the middle finger.
Insert the finger gently into the rectum and feel for a hardened ball of BM (bowel contents). If found, call the doctor.

— The doctor may order an oil enema, such as Fleet's and explain that the impaction needs to broken up manually. Again insert your well-lubricated finger into the rectum, and gently start breaking up the impacted ball so it can be removed or expelled. Despite the care taken, a small amount of bleeding might be seen. Clean the anal area and place a cloth (rung out of ice water) or a small ice pack over the area for a few minutes.

This is an uncomfortable procedure, but once the obstructing BM is removed, your loved one will gain relief. If the discomfort continues for several hours, place a very warm, wet-pack over the area or prepare a warm tub bath. The warm water treatment may be repeated.

Coping with Poor Bladder or Bowel Control

As we grow older, some loss of bladder or bowel control is not uncommon. It is one of the chief reasons for nursing home admissions.

Urologists are usually able to correct or improve the condition with treatment. When incontinence is untreated, the accidental dribbling affects the person's life. She may be afraid to cough, sneeze or laugh heartily. She may drink less fluids and stay home more often because she is embarrassed by accidents. You can help by reminding your loved one to empty her bladder every two to three hours during the day.

A routine should be followed for bowel evacuation. Encourage her to drink adequate fluids and plan meals with more roughage and fruit. She can wear a pad for adequate protection while attending social gatherings. Anyone who wears an indwelling catheter or has a colostomy lives with established routines.

Tips for Care with Bladder Problems

- When a man is incontinent, a newborn disposable diaper may be wrapped around the entire penis and secured with a tape tab. Fold the open end and tape it shut.

- If the man is unconscious or paralyzed, cut a two-inch slit toward one end of a disposable bed pad. Place the pad over the abdomen and pubic area with the absorbent side next to the skin. Slip the penis through the slot and position it in a plastic urinal. The pad will extend under the urinal and protect the bed from accidental spills.

- If someone wears a catheter, keep the drainage bag below the level of the bladder. For wheelchair users, insert a grommet (metal eyelet) through the lower edge of the vinyl chair back. Place an "S" hook through the grommet and hang the drainage bag. Cover the bag when out in public.

  Second method:

  Fasten or tape a heavy clothes hanger to each side across the back of the chair. Aim the hook toward the floor and hang the drainage bag on it. With either method, the bag will not drag on the floor. Cover the bag when out in public.

- Place a terry cloth wristband (purchased or homemade) around the neck of the urinal to prevent irritation to the inner thighs.

- With certain conditions, the doctor may ask the nurse to teach your loved one how to self-catheterize. You should know how to perform a catheterization if necessary. Help him maintain a six hour schedule, keep an accurate intake and output record and be alert for any symptoms of a urinary infection.

Tips for Care with Bowel Problems

- You may give a warmed Fleet's enema by dropping the bag in the bath water during a bath. It may also be warmed by placing the bag in a microwave oven for about 15-20 seconds. Test the fluid on your wrist before giving the enema to be sure it is a comfortable temperature.

- Sprinkle baby powder around the edge of a bed pan to prevent the skin from sticking as the person slips on and off. A lotion may be used instead.

- If a loved one needs a bed pan while sitting in a chair or wheelchair, try reversing the pan's position and slipping the front under first. The pan will support the thighs without cutting into them and is more easily removed.

- Your patient may have difficulty holding the enema solution due to a weak sphincter muscle, or large hemorrhoids. Buy an ordinary rectal tube, attach it to the tip of a disposable enema and deposit the solution higher into the lower colon. Or you may purchase a rubber baby nipple, cut a hole in the end and slip the enema nozzle through it. The nipple works as a plug.

- A bedfast or disabled person who is incontinent may wish to wear underpants. Choose a white cotton knit pair which is one size larger than regularly worn to allow for shrinkage. Open the side seams and stitch velcro strips along each side. The pants are easily put on and removed.

- If a stool specimen has been ordered, try one of these easy ways to collect it:
  - Drape a piece of plastic wrap or plastic bag over the toilet bowl when the seat is raised and tape the edges to the outside of the bowl. Put the seat down, let the stool drop onto the plastic wrap, and with a throw-away plastic knife lift off a specimen. Drop the rest into the bowl.
  - Rinse a bed pan with water, press a large plastic bag into the inside contour of the pan and let the bag drape over the outside. After the bed pan is used for a BM, lift the specimen out and empty the rest into the commode. If a total specimen is required, tie the bag edges together for transporting.

Ostomy Care at Home

The colostomy or ileostomy, a new opening to eliminate bowel contents. may be temporary or permanent. During the hospital stay, the patient will become familiar with the equipment and the daily procedures necessary to manage the ostomy. An ongoing source of support will be the members of the local ostomy association, for they have coped with all the problems. Recent articles in the *Ostomy Quarterly* magazine were written by a man who has had an ostomy for 58 years and by a 100-year old man who has had his ostomy for ten years. He continues to care for a retarded son.

Once home, the goal is to manage the ostomy so that he will be able to continue his previous activities. When well managed, he will evacuate about the same time each day and will avoid unexpected movements. Meals should be served on schedule and the food should be chewed slowly. Through some trial and error, the person should produce a soft stool consistently. One secret is to try new foods one at a time to determine their effect on the stool. Most people with a colostomy do not let it interfere with their daily lives.

Other tips are:

- For the first six weeks, the diet should be slightly constipating. The person should eat smaller servings of fibrous foods, such as corn, celery, coleslaw, nuts, raisins, grapefruit, fried foods.

- To help prevent diarrhea, avoid serving highly spiced foods or raw fruits and vegetables such as green beans, broccoli and spinach.

- Avoid gas forming offenders which include: beer, highly spiced foods, carbonated drinks, cabbage, beans, cucumbers and radishes. Chewing gum, smoking and drinking liquids increases the amount of air swallowed. The product "Beano" among others guarantees to prevent gas formation from beans. Deodorant products can be placed in the pouch.

Care When Taking Medicines

Iron and vitamin supplements will discolor the stool or urine. Depending on whether the ostomy opening is high (small bowel) or lower in the bowel, the tablets or capsules may not have time to be absorbed before being eliminated. Check the drainage bag when a new medication is started. Many medications are available in a liquid or chewable form which will absorb more quickly.

Ostomy Problems and Solutions

- The abdomen may appear smooth when a person lies flat, but on sitting or standing, have creases and lines due to extra weight or weakened muscles which may allow leaks around the face plate of the drainage pouch.

- When the opening (stoma) is first made it will be swollen. After about 6-8 weeks it will shrink to its permanent size. It may not be perfectly round, and if not, a cut-to-fit face plate works best.

- Some people with an ostomy may have the opening high in the colon (ileostomy) and continue to have liquid or semi-formed stools that are harder to regulate. Liquid stools soon irritate the skin around the ostomy and require some type of skin barrier. An ostomy powder is available which absorbs some of the moisture, becomes a sticky gel, and forms a barrier to protect the skin. If stools remain loose, ask the doctor if a bulk-forming product (such as Metamucil) or a medication (such as Lomotil) might reduce the amount of liquid stool.

- An inexpensive substitute for a colostomy irrigation bag is a douche bag. It is sturdier and is about one-third the cost.

- A small emergency kit may save embarrassment. Place a pair of underpants, a small clean cloth or a moist towelette, a small bottle of deodorant and a stoma bag in a shaving kit or makeup case.

Note: Do not use greasy creams, ointments or oil soaps around the stoma (opening.) Use only the products developed for use under the adhesives. In rare instances, a person may develop a mild reaction to a product, and should switch to another. Every problem has a solution and other ostomy users have answers.

MEETING THE BODY'S NEEDS

The selection of food is especially important for the person experiencing the side effects of treatment, such as a sore mouth, changes in taste sensations, severe or chronic nausea, etc.

Certain foods soothe the body and adequate fluids help it renew itself. This chapter discusses how to help meet the body's needs when it is not functioning normally.

Preparing and Handling Food

Aging gradually weakens the immune system, stomach and kidneys which help fight off and control bacteria. Someone coping with a chronic illness such as diabetes, or undergoing medical treatments such as chemotherapy, is especially vulnerable. A food-borne illness (food poisoning) can have serious consequences and may interfere with treatment. To keep food safe, follow these guidelines:

- Refrigerate all perishables. Freeze raw meat or poultry that won't be used in two days.

- Don't thaw foods on the kitchen counter, for bacteria multiply at room temperature. When thawing food in the refrigerator, place a plate under it so raw juices can't drip and contaminate vegetables or other food.

- Wash your hands thoroughly before and after handling food. Wash utensils and cutting boards in hot, soapy water after cutting raw poultry or meat. If you have a choice, buy a plastic board.

- Thoroughly cook raw meat, poultry or fish. Cook eggs until white and yolk are firm. A person with a weakened immune system should be especially careful to eat well-cooked foods.

- Follow directions when cooking in the microwave.

- Freeze or refrigerate leftovers right away, not after cooling on the counter.

- Never leave perishable food out of the refrigerator more than two hours while shopping or serving a meal. Don't take leftovers home. Consider this after a family picnic, church supper, etc.

  Note: Check cans or glass jars for dents, cracks or bulging lids. Make sure the refrigerator is 40 degrees Fahrenheit or lower. The freezer should register 0 degrees or lower.

(From Healthwatch in <u>Aging Magazine</u> 1994)

The public is bombarded with articles on nutrition in magazines and newspapers until most adults have a clear understanding of the body's needs. However, when the body is not functioning normally, less information is readily available. Many caregivers may cope with one or more of the following conditions:

When Someone Has a Poor Appetite or Has Lost Weight

- The appetite is usually best during the morning hours. Prepare a good breakfast or brunch.

- Unless prohibited while taking a medicine, a glass of beer or wine may be given before a meal to increase the appetite.

- Avoid fried foods or foods with a high fat content. These tend to stay in the stomach longer and will result in a false feeling of fullness.

- Unless he is nauseated, encourage the person to make a conscious effort to eat - even if not hungry.

- If he eats very little and feels full quickly, give a supplement. Supplements are formulated to provide high quality nutrition in a compact form. These supplements include: ENSURE, ENSURE PLUS, MERITENE, SUSTACAL, SUSTACAL HC (high calorie.) A supplement may be offered directly from the can or mixed with ice cream, sherbet, frozen yogurt or blended with fruit. Open the can, freeze, and eat the supplement like ice cream. Freezing often improves the taste.

From a handout by Elissa Blackham,
University Hospital, Las Vegas, NV Dietitian

When the Taste Sensation is Altered
(As with Chemotherapy)

- Sweet foods may have less taste while bitter foods taste stronger. Fresh fruits may improve the taste of milk shakes, ice cream, puddings, custards or prepared supplements.

- Foods high in protein, especially red meat, may taste bitter. Substitute fish or chicken. If the person has a problem with these, experiment with recipes that have a more appealing taste to him. You may substitute eggs, cheese, soy products and cured meats such as ham, bacon, sausage or corned beef.

- Marinate meats in soy sauce, sweet fruit juices, sweet wines or cook them with fruit. Foods can be made more flavorful by adding seasonings, such as lemon juice, mint, basil, or any of the newer mixed spice preparations.

• Serve dried beans, lentils and peas to add protein to the diet. Offer protein supplements and try the recipes in a vegetarian cookbook.

Note: As stated in the chapter on Cancer, <u>a high-protein diet during chemotherapy helps the effectiveness of the treatment</u>.

When the Mouth is Sore or Dry
(As with Chemotherapy)

Soft, cold foods such as ice cream, watermelon or frozen fruit bars may feel and taste good when the mouth is sore. Offer apple juice to drink and prepare main dishes which contain a gravy or heavy sauce. Drinking through a straw may make swallowing easier. Liquids or moist foods help a person with a dry mouth. Serve broths, gravies, stews, casseroles and cold cream soups. The person may dunk his food in a liquid, such as coffee, milk, tea or hot chocolate.
(From booklets published by Adria and Ross Laboratories)

When One Has Difficulty Swallowing

• Help him sit in an upright position, or prop with pillows until he is in a near sitting position if lying in bed.

• To make swallowing easier, remind him not to throw the head back, but hold the chin at a natural level.

• Food should be cut into small bites. One should eat about a teaspoonful at a time.

• Alternate food with sips of liquid. Carbonated drinks are better tolerated than water. Liquids may be hard to swallow. Adding a thickener helps. Try a few potato flakes or a commercial thickener. One product is "Thick-It," from Bruce

Medical Supply (800-225-8446) which can be tried as a free sample first. Use a flexible straw.

- Serve foods which have rich flavors, if possible, for they are easier to swallow.

- Plan for a quiet time and less conversation during the meal.

- When the person finishes eating, he should remain upright for about 15-30 minutes to let gravity help the cough reflex. Don't try to stop him if he coughs.

- Try serving ground foods, mashed potatoes/gravy, yams, yogurts, pasta with flavorful sauces, mashed vegetables, fruit sauces. Try supplements, such as Ensure, in regular or frozen form.

How to Help Counteract Nausea

Offer foods that move through the stomach quickly, such as the high-carbohydrate foods: crackers, toast, gelatin and juices.

Carbonated drinks, served cold, may help relieve nausea. Serve one of the following foods as the stomach settles: rice, soft boiled or poached eggs, custard, soda crackers, apple juice, apricot and pear nectars. Cool, clear beverages, lowfat fruit ices, dry toast and crackers may help calm the stomach.

Help Following Episodes of Vomiting:

- Serve salty foods and avoid overly sweet ones.

- Replace the fluids lost by providing clear liquids such as broths, ginger ale and those mentioned above. Use juices to make ice cubes. The person should drink a moderate amount of fluids at mealtime.

- Cooking odors may make a person nauseated. He or she should move to another room or out of doors while you are cooking. Serve more cold foods such as meat, salad, sandwiches, cold soups or desserts with fruit.

- Do not be concerned about balanced meals when the person is nauseated or vomiting. Try to add supplements to the food you prepare, such as adding protein powder or dry milk to increase the protein content of a dish.

Help Following Bouts of Diarrhea

- Prepare smaller portions of low fat foods and serve them more frequently. (Use smaller plates and prepare food attractively.)

- Potassium and sodium have been lost from the body. Serve high potassium foods which are easily digested. These include potatoes, bananas, peach or apricot nectar, fish or other meat.

- Serve peeled, cooked fruits and vegetables without seeds.

- Certain foods may tend to create more diarrhea. Some people may not tolerate milk products. Also to be avoided: greasy, fatty or fried foods, beans, broccoli, corn, onions, garlic, popcorn and nuts.

Help for the Complications of HIV or AIDS

Diarrhea (with poor absorption of food nutrients)

The person may have chronic diarrhea, may develop nutritional deficiencies and eventually will have a loss of weight. If the diarrhea is mild, the watery stools may be reduced by taking a high-fiber supplement, such as ENRICH. He or she should start by taking small amounts to avoid gas formation and bloating. Serve small, frequent meals which are low in caffeine, fat and lactose (milk and cheese). Add a liquid supplement, such as ENSURE PLUS HN.

Painful Lesions in the Mouth

As you prepare the food, omit highly seasoned, acidic or salty foods and those that are dry, sticky or abrasive. Foods that are very cold (ice cream) or very hot (tea or coffee) may cause pain. The person may tolerate both fluids and blenderized foods. Add gravies, sauces and broth to make foods easier to swallow. Many people prefer to drink high-calorie, high-protein liquids (such as ENSURE or ENSURE HN) than to eat solid food.

The doctor may order a diet with increased calories or protein. To add additional calories:

- Use heavy cream, whole or evaporated milk instead of water whenever possible. Add sour cream to baked potatoes, vegetables and fruits.

- Melt butter or margarine on to hot foods such as toast, soups, cooked cereals, rice or vegetables. Spread cream cheese (try adding fruit for flavor) on bagels and toast.

- Use canned fruit with a heavy syrup. Stir fruit into yogurt and put some on cereal, ice cream and other desserts. Use sugar, jelly or honey to sweeten cereal, fruit and toast.

How to Add Flavors to Liquid Supplements

- Open a can of supplement (ENSURE, ENRICH) and place in the freezer. When frozen, eat as ice cream.

- Combine 3/4 cup ENSURE or ENRICH (vanilla) with 1 package of cream of chicken soup mix (instant.) To prepare: Heat the liquid but do not boil. Then add to the powdered soup mix, stir and serve.

- Combine 3/4 cup ENSURE (vanilla), 1 can cheddar cheese soup and 1/2 cup water in a saucepan. Stir, then add 1 teaspoon of worcestershire sauce plus a dash of salt. Heat but do not boil.

- To 1 cup ENSURE or ENSURE PLUS add 1 teaspoon instant coffee powder, 2 tablespoons chocolate syrup and a dash of cinnamon. Stir well to blend.

- To 8 ounces of vanilla flavored ENSURE, ENRICH, ENSURE PLUS or ENSURE PLUS HN, add one of the following and blend:

  1 serving of chocolate drink mix
  1 level teaspoon of instant coffee
  1 tablespoon of powdered butterscotch pudding mix
     (a little brown sugar adds flavor)
  1 heaping teaspoon of malt powder
  1 teaspoon of peanut butter
  1 tablespoon of powdered egg custard mix. Add a little
     vanilla. Blend well, then add a sprinkle of nutmeg.

  The drink may thicken when it is refrigerated. You may substitute a few drops of lemon, orange or almond extract for a different flavor.

These suggestions are taken from the booklet
"Dietary Modification in HIV Disease"
Ross Laboratories, Columbus, Ohio, 433216

Other Suggestions about Food

- Cooked foods may be put in a blender to produce a smooth puree or soup. Add broth for the liquid and season. Examples of dishes that blend well are: chicken with rice, beef with potatoes or ham with red beans.

- Use crushed ice with a frozen fruit juice concentrate to make a "slush."

- If sugar is poorly tolerated, try using the juice from canned fruits (packed in natural juices) as a substitute for sugar.

- As long as the mouth is not sore, sour foods such as lemons, dill pickles or sour pickles may help curb the nausea from the chemotherapy treatment. Dill pickle juice alone stopped one person's chronic nausea.

- An easy recipe for a high protein meat loaf:
  2 pounds of lean ground beef or turkey
  1/2 cup of each - wheat germ, evaporated milk, nonfat dry milk
  Prepare the rest of the meat loaf as usual.
    From Sue Williams, Consulting Dietician, Kaiser Permanente

How to Help Curb the Appetite
(Help control weight)

How to fool the body into thinking it is full when it's not:

- One-half hour before dinner, offer tidbits of raw vegetables with a low calorie dip, fresh fruits and hot spiced tea. These "appetite spoilers" begin raising the blood sugar level, sending impulses to inform the brain that the body has been fed. This process requires about 40 minutes, so that by the time the dinner is served, the person has begun to feel satisfied.

- Other foods that achieve the same result include:
  1/2 cup berries or melon balls, celery stuffed with low fat
    pot cheese and a bowl of consomme
  1/2 cup of plain yogurt, one apple and some
    sunflower seeds
  Assorted raw vegetables, fruit juice over ice
    (in pretty glass)
From an article by Barbara Winkler, describing The Golden Door Spa

  Note: Substitute a mixed spice mixture for salt. Salt is usually added to canned vegetables, even those low in salt content, and to most restaurant dishes. As a people, we tend to ingest more salt than our body needs.

Foods that Can Influence Our Emotions

Several years ago the author of the Southampton Diet Book listed "happy" and "sad" foods. Lists are included for your consideration as you select your menu.

"Happy" foods

Milk, turkey, chicken, cheese, bananas, beef, pineapple and yogurt all contain tryptophan (an amino acid that acts as an antidepressant).
Lean red meat (beef, other game meats - exclude pork), organ meats, whole grains, yeast, wheat germ, green leafy vegetables and brown rice (shell of the rice), which contain the B vitamins and folic acid. Oranges, grapefruits, lemons or limes, strawberries, broccoli, green peppers, spinach, brussels sprouts and cantaloupe contain vitamin C.

"Sad" foods

Sugar (produces "sugar blues"), egg yolks, marbled meats and wheat cereals contain choline which may increase depression. Aged cheese, pickled herring, Chianti, sour cream, beer, ripe avocados and aged beef contain a competitor of an amino acid that helps relieve depression. Lobsters contain GABA (gamma aminobutyric acid) which leads to lethargy. Peas, lentils and chick peas inhibit thyroid activity.

Maintaining Adequate Fluids

Fluids keep the skin moist, the mouth and tongue from feeling sticky, and the body's cells moving and transferring products. The kidneys wash out the end products of metabolism and the bowel eliminates the softer food waste. Without enough water, our body will tell us it is thirsty. Or does it?

Sometimes a person, for whatever reason, fails to drink enough liquids and does not feel thirsty. The 50-60 ounces (6-8 glasses) of fluids needed daily may be taken in juices, soup, Jello, shakes as well as water, milk, tea and coffee. Here are some ways to make drinks more flavorful and interesting:

- Keep water in a pitcher or bottle in the refrigerator. Add a few lemon, lime or orange slices.

- Freeze juices in ice cube trays to serve with drinks. Stick two or three tooth picks in some of the cubes before freezing and serve as popsicles which are welcome if someone is on a restricted fluid intake (limited amount of fluids daily).

- Add a citrus juice to tea (hot or cold) and add honey.

- Serve cold soups (potato, tomato, beet borscht, gazpacho) in hot weather and hearty, hot soups in cold weather.

- Add a small amount of hot chocolate mix to hot coffee, cinnamon to hot chocolate and a few cinnamon candies ("red hots") to hot apple juice or cider before serving.

- Use juice as part of the liquid when making Jello.

- Add ginger ale, 7-up or calorie free, flavored carbonated beverages (such as Free and Clear) to fruit juices for "zing."

Recognizing Symptoms of Dehydration

Your loved one's body is well-hydrated. The intake of fluids and the output of urine seem well balanced. Then he becomes ill and he loses more water that he drinks. The loss of extra water may be due to a severe cold with a cough, a heavy production of sputum, a low grade fever of several days duration or a bout of vomiting and diarrhea. When the body needs more fluids, the person will usually feel thirsty.

Note: How to check if the body needs more fluids:

Gently pinch a fold of skin on the back of the hand between your thumb and forefinger. Release the skin suddenly. If the elevated fold remains and slowly sinks into place, consider that the body needs more fluids. If the skin drops in place quickly, the body appears to be adequately hydrated.

Signs and Symptoms of Dehydration

Several of the following signs and symptoms will be present:
- May complain of thirst.

- The mouth is dry, lining is sticky or tongue is swollen.

- Has dark circles under the eyes or the eyeballs appear sunken.

- The urine is darker in color and smaller in amount.

- The temperature is above normal.

- He is constipated or has lost weight.

- He appears confused or agitated (especially if elderly).

- He eats and drinks very little.

Keeping a Record of Intake and Output

You may believe your loved one is taking adequate liquids every day, but you have noticed several of the symptoms of dehydration. An accurate record of the person's intake of fluids for a few days will provide a clear picture. If the urine output has decreased, you note a strong odor and the color has become dark amber in color, keep a record of the output also.

How to Calculate Intake

Calculate the liquid portion of foods. For instance:
Jello = 3/4 of total (with fruit added = 1/2)
Watermelon = 3/4 of total
Pudding = 1/2 of total

Soup = estimate liquid portion
Ice cream, yogurt, apple sauce, Ensure, etc.= 1/2 of total

Measuring Equipment for the Intake

One easy method is to pour an equal amount of water into a large pitcher, jug or jar each time the person has a drink. Use one that is calibrated with lines for ounces, pints, etc. Total the water and estimate the amount of fluid in the food eaten for 24-hours.

A second method is to fill a measuring cup with the water from a favorite cup or glass to learn how many ounces they hold. Cups may hold from 4-8 ounces and a glass holds from 8-16 ounces. You may place a strip of tape on the outside indicating the ounces. Record all fluids ingested on a sheet of paper and total every 24 hours.

Recording Output

Ask your loved one to void (urinate) into a plastic urinal (from a hospital stay), an old calibrated pitcher or a bedpan. Record the amount of urine excreted. If the person has a watery stool, estimate the amount of water lost. Make a note if the person has been sweating profusely, has been bleeding or has vomited one or more times during the day. Each causes a loss of fluid from the body. Total the output for the same 24-hour period as the intake.

Note: When the output drops below 20-23 ounces (600-700cc) in a 24-hour period, the body cannot wash out all the waste products from metabolism. Calculate the intake and output as accurately as you can and if you suspect the person is dehydrated, notify the doctor.

Chapter Six

HELPING WITH MOBILITY

The person who has lost the ability to walk without assistance, even temporarily, must depend on a wheelchair, crutches, walker or cane for mobility. The caregiver should become acquainted with the mobility aids, adjustments, positioning and the walking procedures to help the user improve his ability to maneuver effortlessly.

Selecting a Wheelchair

A wheelchair conserves energy when the person is too weak to maneuver crutches and is the preferred aid in crowded airports.

- Various models are available. The standard models are heavier, but if one has good balance, a light weight model can be used. A person under five feet tall may use a "hemi" wheelchair.

- Chair seat widths include 14 inches for youth and 16, 18, 19 and 20 inch for adults. When seated, the user needs to allow one (1) inch between arm rest and hip on each side. Keep in mind, the narrower the chair, the easier it is to maneuver through doorways. Chairs have a standard seat depth and back height unless special ordered. The footrest extension length is adjustable.

- Wheelchair options include:
  - **Armrests**

    Removable armrests permit the chair to move close to a table or desk and allow the user to exit the chair sideways, which is a blessing if both legs do not function well. When armrests are removed, the chair becomes lighter and easier to lift into a car or van.
  - **Footrests**

    Removable, side-swinging footrests can be purchased in several sizes and should have heel loops to prevent a poorly-controlled foot from slipping or sliding under the chair.
  - **Leg rests**

    Removable leg rests which elevate, are necessary if the person has a serious problem with swollen feet and legs or if they wear a rigid brace or cast.
  - **Folding chair**

    Most chairs are collapsible so the person has freedom to travel.
  - **Seat cushion**

    A cushion should be used. If the chair is to be used part of the time, an ordinary foam rubber cushion will suffice. But if the person sits in a wheelchair during the hours he is out of bed, invest in a gelatin-filled or other special cushion for wheelchair users. It prevents discomfort from sitting and helps prevent tissue break-down. The physical therapist may suggest the best type of cushion.

Note: One electric wheelchair user who is a polio victim, highly recommends using a genuine sheep skin over the wheelchair seat (with or without a seat cushion.) A washable synthetic sheep skin is also available.

Helping Someone Move Into a Wheelchair

Before helping a person into a wheelchair, always lock the chair's wheels. If he is leaving a bed, place the chair close to the bed, facing the foot. Remember to keep your back straight and knees bent and use thigh muscles as you lift.

- If a person is unable to maneuver and help himself, elevate the head of the hospital bed to protect the lifter's back. In a regular bed, use several pillows to elevate. Standing behind the person's back, reach under the arms and lock both hands in front of the chest. If the person is large, hold firmly under the arms. Ask a second person to grasp both ankles, and on a count of three, lift together and swing the disabled person into the wheelchair. Check *Caring for the Sick* for another easy two-person lift.

- If the person is able to sit alone on the side of the bed, position the wheelchair for him. Lower an adjustable-height, hospital bed until the top of the mattress is slightly higher than the wheelchair seat. Remove the chair's armrest (if you can) and encourage the person to reach for the far armrest. Using upper body strength, he will move over into the wheelchair. A smooth, tapered-edged transfer board is available or may be made, and should be placed between the mattress and chair seat to make the transfer easier.

- If the person is able to stand, swing the footrests aside, and support him as he backs up until both legs touch the seat. Ask him to grasp the armrests, get his body centered, and sit down.

  Note: The wheelchair user may not be centered on the chair seat cushion or may not have the hips resting against the back of the chair. Step behind the chair, reach under his arms and lock your hands across his chest. Lift upward and pull him back in the chair seat. When the body is upright and centered, equal pressure will be exerted on each buttock and his muscles will relax. Check that the knees are the same height as the hips or slightly lower.

An easy technique is to use a bath towel to reposition your loved one. Before he is seated, fold the towel lengthwise and place it across the chair seat with the ends extending over front and back edges. Help him to be seated. Stand behind the wheelchair, use both hands to pull evenly on the back edge of the towel. A small caregiver can move a heavier person without back strain.

> To relieve pressure on the tissue under the hip bones, especially without a special cushion, the patient should rock his body to one side, hold a few minutes, then rock to the other side, hold and relax. Pressure should be relieved every 45 minutes to an hour.
>
> When the person has gained enough strength, the doctor may tell him to do "sitting push-ups." You should know how to do the procedure so you can observe and correct his technique. This exercise should not be attempted until the doctor approves.
> — With chair wheels locked, the disabled person grasps the armrests and pushes down until he can lock his elbows.
> — He depresses the shoulders as he pulls the head and neck upward.
> — He tightens the abdominal muscles, tips the pelvis forward and lifts the hips off the seat.
> Try the lift yourself. It is not easy.

Sally Pryor, in her excellent book *Getting Back on Your Feet* offers these reminders:

- A person sitting in a wheelchair is often treated as if they are deaf, ignorant or stupid. When you notice this happening, draw the the person into the conversation.

- Ask a person in a wheelchair if they need some assistance and how you may give it. Do not insist.

- The brakes on the wheelchair must always be locked when the person is sitting still.

- Tie or wedge the room doors open for easy access. Some narrow doors may have to be removed. Take care that fingers are not scraped as the chair goes through a door.

Note: I returned home from another state with my recently, paralyzed son, and we were greeted at the airport by my husband, Bill, holding a wheelchair. Arriving at the house, we soon realized that Bill had sat in the chair and moved all the furniture out of its way. We also discovered a new ramp had been built out to the patio. What a nice welcome for a discouraged, exhausted son and his mother.

Aids for Walking

Your loved one's daily environment may have been reduced to a room, a house, the view from a car window or a short visit. The ability to lift one foot and place it in front of the other is often regained through determination, patience and continued effort. He or she needs your observations when starting to use a walker, crutches or a cane, for it is difficult to evaluate one's self. Check if the user is standing straight and placing the heel down first as with a normal step. Stand in front where you can observe the movements.

The Use of a Walker

Walkers offer the most stability and demand the least coordination. They are light-weight and are available with or without wheels. Wheeled walkers may have forearm supports for someone who lacks strength in the hands, a seat for resting and brakes. A carry-on-basket or oversize wheels may be added.

Wheel-less walkers are made of light-weight aluminum. All walkers are available in collapsible models for easy transporting. The walker's height must be adjustable and the handlebars should come to the level of the user's elbow crease when he stands with both arms hanging at the side. When standing straight on the walker, the user should not need to hunch his shoulders.

How to Walk with a Walker

The person should place the walker in front of him, with hands on each side, and take two equal steps up to it. Starting with the weaker leg or foot, he places the heels down first and uses a normal walking gait. If he prefers, the aluminum walker can be lifted with each step and moved forward. To climb stairs, the person should use the handrail or use a cane instead of the walker. He should start climbing with the stronger leg and foot which will support and lift his weight. Recheck that a folding walker is fully and securely snapped into place before putting weight on it. I recently saw a rubber-tired model which formed a V when unfolded.

The Use of Crutches

Crutches require much more energy than normal walking. Lightweight, underarm, extension crutches are available. The Canadian crutch extends to the elbow, requires less energy, frees the hands and saves wrist strain. It is also more difficult to master and much less stable. These crutches are generally reserved for long-term users who can bear some weight as they walk, have good stability and want to be more active.

The top of the crutch should almost reach the arm pit, but lacks about two inches (two or three fingers) so the person's weight is not suspended from his armpits. Hand grips should be located at the level of the wrist crease when the arm hangs at the side. This allows the arm to be slightly bent (about a 20-30% angle) when the user holds the hand grip.

Many people walk with crutches when both feet and legs are equally weakened. The person should always try to place the heel down first, as in normal walking, to prevent straining the muscles and to improve his progress. The swing-through-method is a good technique for someone who is still weak from time spent in bed, or an elderly person who needs a slower, safer way of walking to conserve energy.

Swing-through Method

The crutches are placed about ten inches in front of the feet and six to ten inches out to each side in a tripod effect. Place crutches about six inches in front of the person who is weak or elderly. The person may move slower but will save energy. The user starts by placing weight on the stronger foot, as the weaker foot steps forward in a natural heel-first position. The weaker foot should be placed just behind the crutches. Using the crutches for partial support, the patient brings the stronger foot up beside the weaker foot. Crutches are brought forward and he continues walking.

A second technique, the **Step-through Method**, starts as the swing-through method, but the stronger foot passes between the crutches as in normal walking. The weight should be equally distributed on each leg. The crutches are brought forward as walking continues.

A third technique, the **Four-point Gait** is the nearest to normal walking. The person starts forward with the weaker foot, then bring both crutches forward at the same time. The stronger leg and foot will come up alone.

Selecting a Cane

A cane provides stability and offers some relief from weight- bearing. It will deliver about one-fifth the propulsion power of a strong leg. The cane may be a family heirloom or borrowed from a friend. The best choices today are aluminum, have a flat, swan neck (as opposed to the old, round-handled, wood one), and can be purchased with a quad (four- footed) base for better balance. Some canes are collapsible. A larger, foam handle is available for users whose hands are weakened from arthritis. A cane tip with a ball-and-socket joint is also available, so that the person can maintain full contact with the ground.

The user should select a cane whose handle height is at the level of the wrist crease when the arm hangs loosely at the side, or he may buy an adjustable cane. Most people select canes that are too long. The person should place the cane in the hand opposite his disabled or weaker side, and should wear low-heeled walking shoes.

How to Walk with a Cane

Hold the cane in the hand on the stronger side and keep it fairly close to the body. Move the cane forward and bring the weaker (opposite) foot forward until the toes are level with the cane. Then bring the stronger foot up beside it. The person may progress until they can move the weaker foot and the cane (still on the stronger side) forward at the same time.

How to be Seated

Your loved one should walk up close to a chair, turn around and back up until the calf of the "good" leg (or both legs) presses against the edge of the seat. Check to be sure that the body is centered and hold one or both arms as he sits down.

When walking with crutches, the user removes them from under the arms, pairs them together and holds them along the long extensions with the strongest hand. Using the crutches for balance, the person reaches with the other hand to hold the back of the chair, and sits down. The crutches should remain within easy reach.

Note: If the calf touches the seat and presses at a slight angle, it will prevent the chair from being pushed back, and allows the person to see where his rear is heading. When using a walker, the person should turn the walker in the direction of the stronger leg. Holding the walker with one hand, the chair back with the other, he sits down.

How to Stand up Again

Getting up requires more effort. The person should scoot the buttocks toward the front edge of the seat and place the strongest foot under the body. If the calf touches the chair, he will have more stability. The crutches should be placed as when being seated. When the person is not strong enough to push upward, he should place one crutch in each hand. Holding firmly to the long side arms, he leans forward and pushes upward. Another technique is to place the weaker hand on the crutch and the strong hand on the chair seat. The person leans forward and pushes upward. Someone who uses a walker may rise in the same manner.

If someone walks with the aid of a cane, he needs to place his feet apart for a stable base. Leaning forward slightly, he holds the cane in one hand, grasps the armrest and pushes upward.

How to Support and Protect Someone From Falling

A disabled loved one may start to fall as you walk together, or as you help him move to another place. Do not try to stop the fall or try to pull him into a chair. The momentum of his weight can cause you injury. You should use your body to protect his head and body as you ease him to the floor.

During a fall, you should:
- Keep your feet apart and your back straight.
- Pull the person close to you as soon as possible.
- Bend your knees and sink to the floor with him against you.
- Make him comfortable until you can get help to lift him.
- If he is not injured and able to assist, help him rise to a sitting position. Locate a solid chair with a low seat and place it behind the person's back. Brace the chair so it won't slide. Or a chair may be placed against the wall so the person can scoot over to it. When a sofa is near, remove the seat cushion so the the short distance makes it easier to lift

the body onto the couch. He will find the easiest way to get onto a seat.

If someone walks with crutches, he may scoot toward the nearest wall and lean each crutch about elbow length from his body. The crutch tips must be pressed down in the carpet or securely anchored. He can gradually work his body up the wall by gripping the crutches with one hand. The best technique is to pull on the crutches while pushing with the strongest leg. Strong leg muscles will lift the body.

If your loved one cannot lift himself, you must find help. Place him into a sitting position, then use the same basic lifting technique as when helping someone out of bed. The stronger lifter drops to a squatting position behind the person, slips both arms under the disabled person's arms and tries to lock the hands across the chest. A second lifter squats at the feet and grasps both ankles. With backs as straight as possible, both lifters use their thigh muscles to lift the person from the floor.

Tips from Sally Pryor in *Getting Back on Your Feet*:

- When your loved one climbs the stairs, stand at the side so he can use the hand rail. If he uses crutches, stand behind him, with one foot on the stair step below and the other foot one step down. Follow him up the stairs.

- When the person descends the stairs, perhaps the safest position is for you to be at his side, ready to grab the belt or waistband. Offer added support by placing your other hand under his armpit. Or you may stand in front and back down. Keep your center of gravity and your base of support firmly established.

Note: I have a courageous friend, Ruth,who went back to work wearing a long leg cast and had to climb stairs to reach her office. She was able to climb the stairs, but felt very unsteady as she looked down the same long staircase in the evening. After consideration, she sat down and dropped her hips gently from step to step. Her progress was slow but no one was watching.

Chapter Seven

CAREGIVING TIPS, PROBLEMS, PROCEDURES

Although caregivers have common concerns and problems, they are also faced with problems specific to their disabled loved one. Aside from the disability, one may have the weaknesses of age, the complications from a chronic illness and the treatments following a hospital visit. Like a spare drawer in the kitchen which holds "odds and ends," this chapter contains a number of general information tips that do not fit in any special category, but are worth knowing.

Home I.V. Therapy

Antibiotics, pain medications and even chemotherapy agents may be given at home through small, programmable IV pumps. In fact, over 250,000 people have had shorter hospital stays, been able to return to work or have enjoyed their final days at home because of home IV therapy.

When the nurse starts an IV, the sting of a pin prick is tolerable unless the vein is elusive. The real teeth-grinding occurs with the anticipation of the repeated probing of a scarred, often-used vein. To spare a loved one from any more discomfort, ask the doctor, nurse or technician if they will first spray the area with a topical anesthetic to numb the skin.

You may help your loved one and the nurse who starts the IV if you try one of these:

- Ask the person to squeeze a small rubber ball in each hand for a few minutes several times each day. In a short time, the veins should protrude enough that it will be easier to insert the needle.

- When an elderly person has veins that look large, but are very fragile, ask him to let his arm hang down as he opens and closes the hand for a few minutes. If the area is lightly taped before inserting the needle, a tourniquet may not be needed.

- Ask the nurse who will start an IV to call about 20 minutes before she plans to arrive. You will have time to wring a thick wash cloth out of very warm water (as hot as you can tolerate on your wrist or elbow) and place it over the person's inner arm at the elbow. Cover it with a dry cloth and wrap completely with a plastic wrap (such as Saran Wrap). When the wet wrap is removed, the veins will be more visible. If starting an IV has been difficult in the past, you may prepare both arms the same way.

Once the IV has been started, both you and your loved one should check periodically to be sure the fluid is dripping and that the IV fluid has not infiltrated into the tissue surrounding the vein. Although the chance of leaking outside the vein is slim, you should check for the following signs:

> The skin looks puffy beyond the tip of the needle (a round, elevated area).
>
> The person may feel uncomfortable, with aching or a slightly burning sensation in the area.

A quick way to check is to hold a small flashlight against the skin directly over the area. When fluid has not seeped into the tissues, only a small halo will appear around the light. But when an amount of fluid is lying in the tissues, the flashlight's beam will highlight the pool of fluid. If you suspect that the IV has infiltrated, contact the nurse.

Caring for an Indwelling Catheter in the Vein

The doctor may have ordered that a Hickman Catheter be inserted to protect fragile veins from repeated punctures. It is held in place by an internal cuff and one external stitch. Usually the skin site is covered by a transparent dressing whose unique qualities allow perspiration to escape, but keep outside water and bacteria from reaching the skin. Ask the hospital nurse or home care nurse how to care for the catheter, what problems to watch for and whom to call.

Dialysis at Home

A dialysis procedure may be given partially or completely in the home. When a person's kidneys function so poorly that a dialysis is needed, the doctor may place a catheter through the abdominal wall which allows a solution to run slowly into the abdominal cavity. The uremic wastes will either drain out by gravity or be drained in a dialysis center. If this procedure can be used, it allows for more mobility and greater freedom. It is also less expensive. For the sake of a loved one, caregivers can learn to give this type of dialysis at home. The nurse will give careful instructions and will decide when the caregiver no longer needs supervision.

Solving Some of the Problems of Aging

- **Failing Eyesight**
  Minimize shadows with several light sources around the room. Use three-way or higher-wattage bulbs and dimmer switches. Put night lights in hallways, bedrooms, bathrooms and keep stairways well lit. Mark edge of steps with light paint or tape. Use glow-in-the-dark tape around light switches, doorknobs and keyholes. Use sheer curtains to cut the glare from direct sunlight. Try to contrast colors (light objects on dark surface) and use richer colors (clear glass tends to disappear.)

  People with poor eyesight can read more easily on yellow,

non-glare paper. If colored paper is not available, highlight the print with a yellow highlighter. When possible use larger print.

- **Hearing Problems**
If someone has trouble hearing an alarm clock ringing, place a large glass behind it. The glass magnifies the ring.

- **Arthritis**
Change the door knobs, especially on outside doors. Install a lever-type knob. It is easier to use and can be operated by depressing it with an elbow when both hands are full. Loop an 18-inch rope or belt though the refrigerator door handle and fasten the loop. If someone cannot grasp the handle, he can slip his arm through the loop and pull the door open. To further assist opening the door, wedge a wooden spoon/paddle between the rubber seal and the door and gently pry it open.

- **Difficulty in Bending**
Pull a wire hanger into a long, straight shape for a two foot "grabber." The extension will help when something drops or is placed on an inaccessible shelf.

- **Communication Difficulties**
As with aphasia following a stroke, the inability to communicate presents a problem for both of you. A set of 3 x 5 cards with messages hand-printed in large letters may help you understand your loved one's wishes. The cards may read "I'd like more"; "I'm thirsty"; "I'm cold, hot, just right"; "The TV is too loud-soft"; "Did I get any mail?"; etc. Punch holes in the cards and slip them through a large key ring. If necessary, you might draw pictures on the cards for better comprehension. Several companies have designed similar message cards. The person will feel less isolated if understood and though unable to speak he might be able to write.

- **Swelling in the Legs**

  As one grows older their legs may swell during the day. To prevent discomfort or damage to the skin and underlying tissues the person should:

  — Elevate the legs several times a day, so the pooled blood can flow back toward the heart.

  — Always prop the feet up on a stool or low chair when seated.

  — Not stand still in one place for a long period of time.

  — Elevate the feet on a pillow when lying in bed.

  — Eat an adequate amount of protein (a deficiency may cause fluids to seep from the tissues into the circulation) and take a multiple vitamin/mineral supplement.

  — Wear elastic hose to prevent swelling (men's or women's) or use an elastic bandage (if ordered by the doctor).

- **Skin That Itches**

  Itching may occur with or without a rash. Untreated, it disturbs sleep, causes irritability, makes one weary and interferes with pleasure. Try to determine the cause so you can help stop the discomfort.

  — An older person's thinner, more sensitive skin becomes dry. When young, the skin's natural oils lock in moisture, but now moisturizers should be used routinely.

  — Encourage warm baths three times a week, using a soap such as Dove, Tone or Neutrogena. Coat the skin with a moisturizer while it is still damp. Avoid long soaks which tend to dry the underlying tissue. Men may need to be reminded to use a moisturizer.

Note: My 89-year-old aunt, Margaret, has added a small amount of baby oil to every bath water and seldom needs to use a moisturizer. She adds a small squirt of dishwashing soap before letting the water drain and the bathtub has no ring.

If dry skin is not the cause of itching, consider:

- Has the skin been exposed to a new product, such as laundry soap or bath soap?

- Have any new clothes been worn or has a new bed covering been used? Dye or chemicals may be the culprits.

- Have any new medicines been taken, either prescription or over-the-counter drugs?

If you have determined what you believe has caused the rash, and it improves, apply an over-the-counter spray or a cream containing hydrocortisone to control the itching. If the itching is intense and a rash lasts more than one day, check with the doctor. When each new drug is prescribed, ask the pharmacist if the drug's possible side effects may include itching or a rash.

Identity after a Move

When you prepare for the person's move into a nursing home or retirement center, include several framed pictures from past years. Staff members will be reminded of who the new resident is - and who he was. Be sure to include a picture album of family and friends with other familiar items such as a favorite shawl, pillow, coffee cup, ball cap, etc.

Anchoring Dishes

Someone who coordinates poorly may have a problem holding their plate or bowl in place on the table or tray. Slip a sheet of the rubberized mesh (used to open jars) under the dishes.

Homemade Hot Packs and Ice Packs

If the doctor orders hot compresses for a few days, fill a slow-cooker or rice cooker half full of hot tap water, turn to the low temperature setting, and place in the room where the pack will be used. Drop a small hand towel or wash cloth in the hot water. With a fork or tongs, lift the cloth out of the water and hold till cool enough to handle. Be careful not to burn the person as you fold and place the cloth on the skin. As the pack cools, you will have hot water nearby if you need to repeat the process.

To make a moldable ice pack, prepare one of these:

- Saturate a sponge with water, place in Zip-Lok bag and put in the freezer.

- Wring most of the water out of a wash cloth or hand towel, fold to the size needed and place on a piece of foil. Freeze until crystals form and the cloth is still moldable.

- Fill a quart-size, freezer-weight Zip-Lok bag half full of a solution of one (1) part alcohol to three (3) parts water and freeze.

- Use a frozen bag of small vegetables which can be refrozen.

Tip: Do not place an ice pack directly on the skin, but wrap it in a pillow case or washcloth.

Prevent Pressure Sores

One in ten people confined to bed or using a wheelchair may eventually develop a pressure sore. All are preventable. Predisposing factors include immobility, lack of vitamin C, incontinence and inadequate protein intake.

The skin will survive for up to 16 hours with pressure of 200 mm on it, while the muscle tissue under the skin starts to lose its ability to survive with 60-70 mm of pressure after two hours. The amount of weight exerted on the tissue over the hip area, when lying on the back, averages 100 mm. A person who spends most of the time in bed should turn from one side to back to the other side every one and a half to two hours. This keeps the area over the heavy bones (hips, coccyx, ankle, shoulder) healthier. The body can be elevated off the mattress by using a foam "egg crate" pad or an electrically- controlled alternating pressure pad. These stimulate circulation and cushion bony areas.

If an area of skin is reddened, do not start massaging the area. The blood vessels have dilated and need time to return to normal. If you see a whitened area, keep the person off of it and watch to see if it returns to a normal color. If not, discuss the changes with the doctor.

A Deodorizer that Kills Odors

A very effective odor eliminator made from pure citrus fruit, is finally available in drug stores. It was formerly named Citrus II when sold in hospital supply stores. Labeled Citrus Magic, it is packaged in a seven-ounce, non-aerosol can. One or two short sprays destroy all odors in a room, so a can lasts for months.

Cleaning the Mouth

Try using a cold Coke to clean the mouth after vomiting. It cuts phlegm, has a pleasant taste and is safe to swallow.

To remove blood from the mouth, mix a solution of 1/2 hydrogen peroxide and 1/2 ginger ale and apply with a swab.

Swab the mouth with a natural enzyme, papaya juice, which is found in health food stores. It will remove most of the debris and does not injure the mouth. Rinse the mouth with water.

For mouth lesions that give off a foul odor, irrigate regularly with a mild solution of baking soda and lukewarm water. Use an ear syringe to reach all areas of the mouth. The doctor may order another wash, such as 1/2 hydrogen peroxide and 1/2 an astringent mouthwash. Check with the doctor before using mouthwash.

Dry, Burning Eyes

As we age, our eyes may produce less lubrication, appear reddened, and "burn." Use drops of "synthetic tears" solution, or a normal saline wash daily. Wring a washcloth out of very warm water, fold and place over the eyes to help relieve irritation. If the area around the eye appears swollen, reddened, warm to the touch or has any drainage, call the doctor.

Helpful Tips

To clean up spills or to clean the bathtub while sitting down or from a wheelchair, use a child's broom and mop.

Move linens, dishes and personal items down to chair level to make it easier for a disabled loved one to help while seated.

To remove a beard easily, apply a mild skin lotion, wait five minutes, apply a regular shaving cream or soap to the softened beard and use a safety razor.

When an arthritic hand aches from exposure to cold air, slip on an oven mitt. It makes a warm glove, is washable and easily removed.

Use a vinyl apron when someone has difficulty feeding themselves. You may make one from clear plastic material or use a flannel-backed tablecloth material. One nursing home uses a long, rectangular bib of attractive terry cloth backed with plastic. It fastens with velcro and washes easily.

Mouthwash has many uses:

- Rinse an emesis basin (used for vomiting) after it has been used.

- Rinse dentures before placing in the mouth.

- Rinse a bedpan after it has been used.

- Put a small amount on a wet cloth and wipe a plastic chair or floor after accidental voiding or incontinence.

- Put on an old toothbrush to clean under the nails.

A wipe-off bulletin board has many uses:

- Keep reminders to call the doctor, replace supplies, the time a visitor is expected, or to find something your loved one wants.

- Record intake and output measurements and if a 24-hour total has been ordered, record the total.

- Write goals. For instance, "John plans to walk down the hall today and eat lunch on the patio."

- Check any lesions or any condition which changes from day to day. For instance: "A reddened area is 3/4 inch yesterday, but enlarges to just over an inch today, has elevated and is warm to the touch."

An easy way to wash the genital area:

Place a loved one on a bedpan after applying a few drops of lotion or baby oil around the rim. Fill a container with warm, soapy water and pour over the genitalia. Follow by pouring clear, warm water to rinse thoroughly. Remove the bedpan and wipe the area with a towel. Dust the groins with baby powder.

Gift Suggestions.

When friends or loved ones wonder what gift to give a disabled loved one, you may suggest:

- A special dish or meal delivered once a month.

- A comfortable house dress, loose shirt, sweat suit, house slippers.

- Several hours of relief caregiving or an offer to accompany the person for treatment, to a park, movie, shopping or a special event.

- A book of humor or a video of a comic movie.

- Make plans and provide tickets for a special event in the future.

- A number of lessons for a hobby they enjoy.

- Plan a party with old friends of the loved one.

Note: This list of gifts might please a busy caregiver as well. Two books of humor, written by Allen Klein, are *The Healing Power of Humor* and *Quotations to Cheer You Up When the World is Getting You Down*. He writes to help one survive the not-so- funny stuff we confront in our lives, and speaks from personal experience. You may contact Allen Klein at 1034 Page Street, San Francisco, CA, 94117. Cost per book is $12.95 complete.

Enjoyable Activities

The hours, despite television, may seem endless for someone who is less mobile and tires easily. Consider these ideas for variety, enjoyment, relief from boredom and loneliness:

- **Purchase an inexpensive camera.** The person may take pictures of friends who visit, record the growth of children and capture the changing outdoor scenes. Display pictures on a large bulletin board and hold in place with decorative tacks.

- **Make a spice garden.** With seeds, plants and a bag of potting soil any bowl or pan becomes a pot. A small pot of herbs or plants make a departing gift for a visitor.

- **Share hobbies with others.** A busy neighbor's child can be taught to knit, sew, hand-tool a belt, pot a plant, tie a fishing fly or make bread - whatever your loved one enjoys doing.

- **Phone a friend daily.** She may call several of her elderly friends every day for a few minutes conversation. The calls also verify that the others are OK. She might offer to contact an organization's members about a special event or to take a survey.

- **Practice basketball or horseshoe shots.** Buy a child's inexpensive foam ball and hoop set or a rubber horseshoe set. The exercise will improve mobility in the arms and shoulders. These games can be shared with others.

- **Give them a gift of music lessons.** My 87 year old aunt, Sara, has been learning to play a dobro and a guitar during the past few years. She has joined a group of non-professional musicians, who fill requests to play at nursing homes and elsewhere. When asked, she will recite her original, light-hearted poetry. She spends many happy hours practicing and has discovered an unknown talent.

- **Record music and TV programs for others.** An old turntable and a cassette player can be combined to make new tapes of old records. TV programs can be videotaped for those at work.

- **Complete picture albums.** Assembling and sorting pictures of the family is time consuming, but worth the effort. Everyone will enjoy and treasure their family history. Decorate and personalize the album covers.

- **Contact a school or college and offer to tape the text books needed by their blind students.**

- **Offer to keep an animal, bird or plants when the owner is out of town.**

Money Making Ideas

I have included this brief segment for you to consider, have fun discussing and possibly find a project that might be marketable. When one creates something that others may value, his sense of accomplishment is more satisfying than money. Especially for someone with limited opportunities. I have listed three simple ideas that found a market plus several suggestions.

One day I visited a fortune cookie bakery and watched the ladies deftly fold the flat cookies as soon as they were baked. Once in a while, one would be misshapen or poorly folded and would be thrown into a separate bin. Later a large sack was filled with these rejects, labeled "Misfortune Cookies," and sold for one dollar. The owner had made even mistakes profitable.

A friend, Virgil, started a business that produced kits, filled with materials to make a dulcimer. As the business grew, so did the pile of small scraps of beautiful wood. The owner offered a bonus to the employee with an idea for using the scraps. The winner made a small boomerang, hinged so it could be folded and placed in a child's pocket. Boy scouts were asked to take them to the park and fly them. The boomerangs became so popular that extra wood was needed to keep up with the demand.

My cousin, June, designed beautiful crocheted doilies, scarfs, table-cloths etc. One day she wrote her favorite thread company and asked if they might have a use for unusual crochet designs. They were interested and today she is planning her fourth small booklet of designs for the company. They are sold in K-mart stores.

For your consideration:

- Prepare a kit of ready-cut materials, decorations, thread and glue for young people to make small, furry animals, pillows, belts, ball caps, etc. Place on consignment in local stores.

- Make small, triangled bean bags, personalized with a child's name, by using scraps of fleece or fake fur material. Would make a safe toy in the house.

- Place an ad offering to use a family's scraps of material to piece a quilt top for them. The finished top, plus batting and lining could be quilted by computer and would make a personal keepsake.

- Place an ad offering lessons. For a small fee, the person might teach cooking, baking, sewing, music, a foreign language or other skills. They might tutor a student for busy parents who may not have the time.

- Contact a local florist or one who supplies hospital gift shops and offer to supply small, ornate pots filled with a mix of small green or flowering plants. They might match the wholesaler's price and provide healthy plants, attractively decorated.

Chapter Eight

CANCER

Cancer has touched most of us sometime during our lifetime — perhaps more than once. As a relative or friend, we have felt helpless while a loved one fought to survive. Though still one of our greatest killers, more victims do survive today. They remain at home during treatment and cope with the side effects. This chapter discusses thoughts about cancer, the common side effects of treatment and offers suggestions for the caregiver to help minimize these side effects.

"Cancer is not a sentence, it is just a word."
Bernard S. Siegel, MD
Love, Medicine & Miracles

Some Thoughts About Cancer

When you decide not to tell a loved one that they have cancer, the secret initiates a web of false reassurances which will keep his or her pain and fear encapsulated. Only with the very old, very young or the too emotionally fragile is the secret worth the cost.

Secrecy robs the person of others' support, forcing him to survive alone with his anger, fears and denial - for one always instinctively knows. Each participant believes that he protects the other, hoarding words forever unspoken.

Never underestimate the resilience of the human spirit. From moments of crushing fear and hopelessness, it can soar with determination and hope.

Practice the art of listening. Use the simple phrases, "I'm here if you need me," "Have you considered —?" and "I understand." Add the reminder, "We're in this together."

Following an unexpected family crisis, the emotional timetables of those involved often clash. One person needs to talk, another seeks privacy for introspection, while a third, feeling overwhelmed, shuts the fearful situation out of his mind for the moment. Each one deserves the chance to come to grips with the situation - and each one will. Patience and understanding are often the first emotions to be tested.

Hope must survive. When we are caught up in statistics, our unique and individual qualities are forgotten. Ignored are the personal strengths, the individual reactions to treatment and the strong survival instincts forged through past experiences. Most of us are not just an average statistic. We also have a faith in tomorrow - plus a "bit of luck."

The person with cancer and his caregiver should become questioners, seeking answers from medical experts. A list of questions for the doctor should include:

- Have you had extensive experience treating this kind of cancer?

- Whom would you recommend for a second opinion?

- What new research is being done on this type of cancer and where is the nearest Cancer Research Center?

- If it is agreed that treatment will be given in our home town, what other types of supportive treatment do you encourage?

- How do you feel about the value of imagery, nutritional supplements and other holistic approaches, along with conventional treatment?

- What are the odds that this cancer can be put in remission?

There is no room for "half-hearted" approaches. The fight must be fought from the moment the person with cancer chooses treatment. He needs unwavering support from his caregiver and loved ones. He must follow the doctor's orders if his chance for recovery is to be maximized. In one study, as many as 85% of patients taking potentially life-saving chemotherapy pills did not follow the doctor's instructions.

Love and laughter are healers and the body responds. Consider hugs, happy memories and light-hearted laughter as your contribution toward a loved one's treatment.

Someone must remain objective and confident while a loved one wages his valiant battle with cancer. You have volunteered, and you cannot drop your anger and anxiety on his overburdened shoulders. Find your support from understanding friends.

Celebrate small successes: a tumor is smaller, the blood count has improved, a number of short hairs can be seen on a bald head or your loved one is hungry again.

Find beauty in everyday surroundings and celebrate each day of your lives. It will make the bad days easier to survive - for you know they are transient.

Give your loved one the freedom to make his own decisions. You may walk beside him, never having walked in his shoes, and still appreciate the daily struggles and successes. The fight is his, but he is not alone.

Choosing the "best" doctor available to you is probably the single most important decision to be made. The doctor should be highly qualified and have the ability to establish an easy communication. Your loved one has the right to receive clear, direct answers and to be given choices. The time devoted to selecting the doctor is time spent productively.

In the United States, Cancer Research and Treatment Centers share information and use the latest treatments. Each may specialize in one area of research. Unless the doctor stresses that immediate treatment must be started, the person usually has time to seek a second opinion. Once the choice of treatment is made, it may be given near home.

Coping with Cancer

Everyone hears the same diagnosis and each responds in his or her own way. A person copes with a difficult situation in the same way he has survived other problems in the past. Whether scared, angry, impulsive, denying, stoic, or calm, he is courageously trying to understand and accept the present situation.

Janet, a registered nurse diagnosed with cancer, was a "good patient." Her feelings of frustration, fear and loneliness were kept secret, as she told herself that she had everything under control.

First, the specialists did not agree on the best treatment for her. The X-ray technician visited with others, while she faced her first treatment, uncovered, cold and alone. She was just another patient receiving 33 treatments. No one knew her first name and she began to feel that she was not a whole person - just body parts to be treated.

When had she lost control? Soon her control became the "mask" she presented to others. Behind it, she was dealing with her cancer in many different ways: worried, uncertain how to act, afraid and alone. With wry humor, she realized that she didn't have to worry about getting cancer anymore.

She found help from others. One perceptive doctor took time to discuss her feelings. A clinical nurse in psychiatry asked her to draw a picture of herself with cancer. She recognized her attitude about treatment in the sick-looking animal with a tear in its eye and darkened organs. She asked another patient,

"Does the radiation make you feel like your teeth are loose?"

"Yes, you too?" she replied and they laughed together. The doctors had discounted her complaints. She accepted, but did not understand her extreme mood swings. With other patients she removed her "mask," for she was no longer alone.

She survived and returned to nursing. She helps other cancer patients live with their fears and denies her own. She helps by listening, discussing their conditions and encouraging them to trust their doctor's decisions and treatment. You can do the same.

Treatment for Cancer

The goal of most cancer treatment is to destroy the weaker, irregular, overgrown cancer cells with little injury to the stronger, well-formed normal cells. Fast-growing cancer cells require more protein and other nutrients, so the normal cells may be robbed of them. At a time when extra protein and calories are needed, the person with cancer may lose his appetite, have altered taste sensations or find eating difficult with a sore mouth. He may experience bouts of vomiting and diarrhea.

You, the caregiver, must try each day to find foods that are nourishing and appealing. Supplements such as Ensure, instant breakfasts and other balanced, complete meals can be frozen like ice cream, blended with fruit, malt, ice cream or seasoned with various flavors. These may be taken between meals for extra nourishment. If meats taste "bitter" during chemotherapy treatment, add pineapple, peaches or sweet and sour sauce. Check Chapter 5 for more information.

<u>Remember, good nutrition makes cancer cells more susceptible to the drugs prescribed for chemotherapy treatment</u>.

As this book is being written, four types of treatment are most frequently being used:

- Radiation from X-ray or cobalt

- Chemotherapy with various combinations of drugs

- Synthetic hormones or hormone suppressants

- Biologicals which help restore the immune system

Most treatments have side effects. Some people have such mild effects that they are able to continue working and caring for their families. Some have one or more of the unpleasant effects of a particular treatment. They respond by taking medicines to control symptoms, eating nourishing food and getting adequate rest. A few people may experience some miserable episodes.

The side effects of two treatment regimes, radiation and chemotherapy are discussed in this chapter. Suggestions are offered for supportive caregiving.

Radiation Therapy

Though temporary, some mild skin changes may develop over the treated area. The skin may appear dry, uneven in texture or reddened (sunburn effect). As treatments continue, the area may become moist.

- If the skin is dry, use a small amount of mild soap and cleanse gently. Rinse well with warm water. Pat dry. Relieve any itching with cornstarch, or lanolin. Pay attention to the skin folds in the treated area.

- If skin becomes moist, do not use any soap. Rinse with lukewarm water only. Pat dry. Apply antibiotic or other creams as prescribed by their doctor. Treat the skin very gently.

Side Effects of Radiation Treatment

Treatment to the Head and Neck Area

The mucous membranes inside the mouth may swell, an ulcer might form or you may note a little bleeding. The mouth may be dry from the decreased saliva production and may feel "tight" to the person. Loss of hair is not uncommon. The brain may hold a small amount of extra fluid.

- Remind him to drink water frequently during the day.

- Do not serve very hot, very cold, highly spiced, rough, course foods or citrus fruits. He should not use tobacco.

- An artificial saliva solution will relieve a dry mouth, and lip moisturizers help.

- The doctor will describe exercises which will keep mouth muscles supple.

- Wigs are inexpensive and are great morale boosters.

- Notify the doctor if you see a change in coordination, speech or alertness from the previous day. Also report if you see white spots in the mouth or note an odor from drainage.

- The person should rinse the mouth frequently, using a mouthwash the doctor recommends, after meals and at bedtime.

Treatment to the Esophagus and Chest Area

The trachea (windpipe) may become dry and irritated and the esophagus may swell. The person may find swallowing painful, have repeated coughing episodes and learn that taking a breath is uncomfortable.

- He may not eat to avoid the discomfort of swallowing food. If so, notify the doctor. A topical anesthetic or a medication for pain will be ordered. Give 30-45 minutes before meals. Ask the doctor if it is safe to take an antacid, when needed. Ask which cough suppressants are most effective.

- Offer supplements between meals. Keep fresh water nearby. Remind him to drink a full glass when he is free of pain and try to sip fluids often.

- Keep a vaporizer going near your loved one. Move it from room to room with him. Discourage smoking.

- Notify the doctor if breathing becomes more difficult or a fever develops.

Treatment to the Abdomen

Four side effects that might occur are nausea, vomiting, diarrhea, and cystitis.

- The doctor will order a medication to help control nausea and vomiting. Offer soda crackers, melba toast, mild fruit juices or tea.

- Keep the door shut when you are cooking and use the vent fan. Place a towel over a used basin or bedpan to hide offensive odors.

- Freshen the mouth by rinsing with a mouthwash recommended by the doctor.

  Note: A dietitian suggested that my son try eating a dill pickle or sipping a small amount of the juice to stop the chronic feeling of nausea. It worked.

- If diarrhea develops, ask the doctor for a medication (which will also stop cramping).

- Wash the skin after each bowel movement. If the anal area looks red or hemorrhoids develop, help your loved one sit in a tub of warm water above the hips for 30 minutes. Test with your elbow.
  A second method for relief: Wring a soft washcloth out of warm water, fold and place against the anal area until it cools. Repeat several times.

- Encourage liquids at room temperature to replace lost fluids.

- If the person develops the symptoms of cystitis (sense of urgency, frequent voiding, a burning sensation), insist that they start drinking a glass of water or other liquids every two hours to help "flush" the bladder. Check the color and odor of the urine. Notify the doctor if discomfort and frequent voidings continue. Do not force fluids if the doctor has ordered that fluid intake be restricted.

Note: Many patients complete the series of treatments with few side effects. If he is uncomfortable, notify the doctor. Once treatment is completed, the side effects disappear in a short time.

Chemotherapy Treatment

Patient's Comments:
"Taking chemotherapy is only a temporary way of life."
"I have not lost control of my life."
"I know my real enemy is the cancer, not the chemotherapy."
"For the short time it's bad, it's very bad, but when it's not,
 it's bearable."

Side Effects of Chemical Therapy

The most common side effects involve the skin and the GI tract, because these cells divide so rapidly. The other system most affected is the immune system.

Hair follicle cells are vulnerable to chemicals for 90% are in the active growth stage all the time. The drugs may create thinning or complete baldness. Low doses of drugs cause the hair to break off, and high doses will cause it to fall out. The loss usually becomes noticeable 2-3 weeks after therapy starts and the hair may start to grow again between treatments.

- In an effort to prevent hair loss, a soft rubber tourniquet, an inflatable cuff or an ice cap may help with certain temperature-sensitive drugs. These aids are not used if the drugs need to reach the scalp. Most people accept the temporary hair loss and buy a wig in the color they choose.

- Special care for the hair includes:
  — Use a mild, protein-based shampoo and conditioner to help keep hair cells nourished.
  — Do not use a hair dryer, electric rollers, hair clips, elastic bands or barrettes.
  — Avoid hair dye, permanents and harsh hair spray.
  — Use a wide-tooth comb and sleep on a satin pillow case.

  Note: Buy a wig, caps or scarves before the hair starts to fall out. The American Cancer Society has a "Look Good - Feel Better" program designed especially for people in treatment. For information call 1-800-395-LOOK. When the hair starts to grow back, it may be a slightly different color or texture.

- The drugs may act on the skin and nails. They may produce redness, raised wheals (welt), itching, acne-appearing areas, discolored nails or bronze-colored areas of the skin. Report any changes you see to the doctor. Note the onset, the location and the severity of the reaction. The doctor may order a cream such as hydrocortisone or may prescribe a bath with some baking soda added.

  Note: Your loved one's resistance is lowered during treatment. Any infection should have prompt treatment. The first symptom of an infection may be a low-grade fever (100 degrees). If a break in the skin becomes swollen and reddened, notify the doctor.

- Cells in the GI tract divide rather quickly (within 24 hours), and most drugs used in chemotherapy will produce some adverse reactions. Symptoms may include a loss of appetite, nausea, vomiting, swollen membranes lining the mouth and esophagus, diarrhea or constipation.
  — The loss of appetite must not be ignored. Fatigue and altered taste sensations may influence an interest in food.

Medicines to stop nausea or pain should be taken 30-40 minutes before meal time.

— The appetite is usually strongest in the morning. Prepare a high-protein, high-calorie breakfast since one-third of the daily requirement should be eaten in the morning.

— Encourage him to eat even if not hungry. Frequent snacks throughout the day may be easier to get down than three regular meals. It may help to withhold fluids during the meal.

Try not to nag until a meal becomes an ordeal.

— Do not serve gas-forming foods (salads, cabbage, broccoli) or any food that seems to upset his stomach. Do not serve fried foods since these tend to create a full feeling.

— Cover pans and serving dishes to control odors and remove any unpleasant sights such as an emesis basin.

— People often eat more if they have company.

Note: A brief exercise, a short walk or a glass of wine if the doctor approves, taken about 30 minutes before the meal will stimulate the appetite.

Include protein-rich foods, such as yogurt and peanut butter as snacks during the day. The American Cancer Society has a booklet containing high protein/high calorie recipes.

Put drinks or supplements in non-metal containers and keep them cold. Some people have a metallic taste during chemotherapy, and the sight of a metal serving piece may upset them.

• Nausea may vary from mild to severe. A bout of nausea and vomiting often occurs 3-4 hours after the chemotherapy was given. It may continue, intermittently, for as long as 72 hours.

— To prevent or minimize this reaction, the doctor will

order an anti-emetic (anti-nausea) drug, such as Reglan, 30 minutes before the chemotherapy. It should be continued for the next 24 to 48 hours or longer. Some people have found that eating a light snack such as toast or crackers before treatment helps, others prefer to fast.

— During the first few days of chemotherapy, the person should take small drinks of liquids frequently until he has consumed a large amount.

— During chemotherapy, hard candy or breath mints may minimize alterations in taste and help prevent nausea.

— Good mouth care will help remove the taste of chemotherapy.
  Some people eat popsicles and tart foods, others eat light meals, such as soup with crackers.

— The nausea or vomiting can be improved by practicing progressive muscle relaxation, self-hypnosis or positive imagery. You may try music or other types of distraction. Relaxation and distraction often help, especially before a scheduled treatment, when anticipation and dread can be upsetting.

• Lips, tongue and hard palate sometimes become sore and tender. Soreness may start one to two weeks after chemotherapy is given, and may last another 2-3 weeks. Ask the doctor, before treatment, if one of the drugs being given has this side effect. If so, remind your loved one to give his mouth a careful cleaning and rinsing four or more times each day.

— The doctor may order a medicine or may approve a mouthwash such as water mixed with baking soda (1/2 teaspoon to a cup of water). Do not use lemon/glycerin swabs or commercial mouthwashes which usually contain alcohol.

— He should use a soft-bristle toothbrush and fluoride tooth paste. Unless he has pain or bleeding, he may floss with unwaxed dental floss at bedtime. Petroleum jelly or lip balm will help keep the lips moist, and an artificial saliva solution will provide moisture for a dry mouth.

— Be sure dentures fit. If they might cause blisters, remove them until the mouth heals or use only at mealtime.

— Encourage the person to stop smoking and to avoid alcohol.

Note: If the mouth becomes very painful, the doctor will order an analgesic (painkiller) medication. Observe for white, cheesy-looking patches, mouth ulcers or shiny, creamy-white raised areas in the mouth. If found, notify the doctor.

When the throat and the esophagus are involved, the person will feel that they have a lump in their throat. Encourage them to keep drinking fluids frequently.

• To prevent heartburn, the person should eat small, frequent meals, avoid hot, spicy foods, alcohol or smoking. He should sit up for at least an hour after eating. Encourage him not to bend or stoop. If frequent heartburn becomes a problem, ask the doctor which antacids may help.

• A sign of diarrhea is three or more watery stools, often accompanied by abdominal cramping or distension. Diarrhea may begin within 24 hours after chemotherapy drugs have been given. Some drugs are greater offenders than others. Try the following:

— Serve low-fiber foods such as bananas, rice, applesauce or mashed potatoes. Avoid raw vegetables, fruits, whole grain breads or beverages that stimulate or irritate the GI tract.

— Offer a lactose-free (no milk) supplement if he has difficulty eating food.
— Add a pinch of nutmeg to foods to help slow the GI peristaltic movements.
— Ask the doctor if you may give an over-the-counter drug (anti-diarrhea) following each loose stool.
— Protect the skin around the anus with vaseline or A&D ointment.

- Some chemotherapy drugs are known to cause constipation. It may occur 5-8 days after treatment. Give a stool softener daily, increase the bulk in the diet and encourage more fluids. Serve fruits (apple juice, prunes, etc.) which are natural laxatives and offer warm beverages. If none of these measures work, call the doctor.

Most people who receive chemotherapy have a short period after the treatment when undesirable side effects may develop - some more serious than others. The side effects disappear as the person's strength is regained. Hair loss is common, but many of the side effects listed above never occur. A chronic loss of appetite, exhaustion and insomnia are most patients' longer-term complaints. A chronic tiredness greets the person in chemotherapy each morning.

It saps his or her energy and the ability to think. Mornings are the worst, so offer breakfast, but try to plan activities for later in the day.

Treatments of Effect on the Immune System

The immune system has rapid cell reproduction, so most chemotherapy drugs cause some bone marrow depression. The white blood cell, red blood cell and platelet counts are lowered. Neutrophils, a type of leukocyte white cell, are the body's first line of defense as they destroy invading microorganisms. The white and red cell counts are lowest about 8-12 days after chemotherapy, and should return to the normal range in 14-18 days. This is often a reason for the 3-4 week separation between chemotherapy drugs being given.

Special Precautions During Chemotherapy

- Wash your hands often and thoroughly with soap. Use friction and rinse well.

- Ask people with colds to keep away during this time.

- Both you and your loved one should watch for early signs of an infection. A low grade fever (100-101 degrees), dry, non-productive cough, redness or pain in an area not previously affected, may be signs of an infection and should be reported to the doctor promptly.

- Keep fresh flowers or live plants away from anyone getting chemotherapy. Stagnant water or potting soil may harbor infectious organisms. Serve cooked vegetables and fruits rather than fresh.

- If possible, avoid giving enemas, harsh laxatives or inserting suppositories. If an enema or a suppository is ordered, use a lubricant and insert gently.

- Use an electric razor during treatment.

- Report any nosebleeds, bleeding or black-appearing (tarry) stools. When the platelet count is lowered, there is an increased risk of bleeding.

- When the red cell count drops, the body has fewer cells to transport oxygen, so the person receiving chemotherapy may feel fatigued, look pale and be short of breath at times. They should pace themselves and take frequent naps. You should not rush them.

Note: When the immune system is depressed, antibiotics will be given to treat any infections. Many of the normal "good" bacteria are destroyed, leaving women more vulnerable to vaginal fungus infections. While taking antibiotics, a woman should eat yogurt (or take liquid acidophilus,) cut down on sugar and eliminate cheese, beer, wine, vinegar and bread from her diet. She should avoid deodorized tampons, change sanitary napkins often and switch to cotton panties.

Coping With Cancer Pain

Pain is the first word associated with a diagnosis of cancer. This was one of our first concerns when our teenage son was diagnosed with Hodgkin's Disease. During the next six years as he fought his disease, however, he was relatively free of pain. He had one episode of post-operative pain, some burning pain during a short bout of shingles, and general aching when he was out of remission. As soon as he started chemotherapy treatment, the aching stopped.

Pain can be broadly described as:

- Somatic pain which may be dull, sharp, aching or a combination and varies from mild to severe in intensity. In general, this pain can be well controlled when the cause is removed or treated. The pain responds well to analgesics (pain-killing) medicines.

- Neuropathic pain which may be burning, shooting or tingling as with shingles. This pain does not respond as well to analgesics and may require other treatment.

As a caregiver, reassure your loved one that pain can and will be controlled and that he will be free of misery. The doctor needs accurate information in order to prescribe the correct drug and dosage. You have an obligation to believe the complaints of pain for it is a subjective experience. The person in pain must:

- Pinpoint the location

- Describe the pain (using descriptive words)

- Rate the intensity of the pain on a scale of one to five. Check the descriptions of pain on page 27.

Again, let me stress that your loved one's pain will "use up" the pain medication and he will not become addicted. If the pain medication takes more than 30 minutes to start easing the pain, never stops the pain completely or causes side effects, notify the doctor. The medicine has not been effective. Sometimes a pain reliever will be ordered for a specific time with a second drug ordered to prolong or increase the effect of the first. Both drugs should be given at the time ordered. With some conditions, a "ceiling effect" can be reached, which means that increasing the dose of pain reliever will not necessarily provide more relief. The doctor is aware of this and needs an accurate feedback of information from your loved one and you.

Note: Many doctors and nurses who work with hospice patients are very knowledgeable and experienced in the newest combinations of medications and techniques for control of pain. The correct combination of medicines can free the person from pain so completely, that he or she may be able to participate in daily activities with loved ones and friends. The person remains awake, alert and capable of making decisions. If your loved one's doctor has not found a regime which controls his pain adequately, consider asking for a consultation with a doctor experienced with hospice patients.

Most pain can be controlled with pills taken by mouth, which permits the person in pain to play a part in his care. Medicine may be ordered around the clock, instead of as needed, for studies have shown that less medication may be required. Rectal suppositories may be ordered if medications cannot be taken by mouth. A medicine may be given by injection or the doctor may order an infusion pump to provide a continuous medication for the patient-controlled relief of chronic pain. The doctors (and hospice nurses) will adjust the medications to the severity of the pain.

Some drugs, such as morphine, may have side effects. These include constipation, nausea and sedation. The sedative effects usually disappear after a few days of therapy. Nausea may occur alone or may be accompanied by vomiting. The side effects may be treated with antiemetics, such as Compazine or Reglan.

Constipation frequently becomes a problem during treatment and, if morphine or other opiates are ordered, will usually continue. Some nausea and vomiting may be related to constipation. The usual measures such as exercise, adequate fluids, bulk-containing foods, prune juice, etc., may not be effective and the doctor may order a combined laxative and stool softener, such as Senokot-S, which no longer requires a prescription. Doses of the laxative/stool softener may be adjusted so as to not cause diarrhea.

The pain of cancer may originate from the various changes in the body, but it is always modified by the mind. The mind is influenced by past bouts with pain, the method one chooses to cope with a crisis, the person's mental stability and the emotional support offered by others. Without relief from acute pain, the person can concentrate on little else. With general relief, psychological interventions may allow the effect of pain to be reduced.

- **Biofeedback**
  Trains the person to relax specific tight muscles and will help control insomnia and even nausea. While not controlling pain, biofeedback contributes to a person's ability to gain control over his pain.

- **Hypnosis**
  The response to pain is influenced by the depth of the trance. Not all pain responds to hypnosis, but many people are helped regardless of the depth of the hypnotic trance.

- **Counseling**
  Working with a counselor can help one to change attitudes which are detrimental, to gain a better understanding and

acceptance of life and to develop a higher self-esteem. As a result he may feel more highly motivated.

- **Hospice**

  When a person enters the hospice program, it has been observed that the control of pain improves significantly. In hospice, priority is given to psychosocial and spiritual issues. The family and others involved are offered support as well as the patient. Nurses skilled in evaluating and controlling pain are key members of the team effort, and the person regains a sense of security and independence.

The Texas Cancer Council ended their Guidelines for Treatment of Cancer Pain with "A Bill of Rights for People With Cancer Pain."

> *I have the right to have my pain believed by health professionals, family, friends and others around me.*

> *I have a right to have my pain controlled, no matter what its cause or how severe it might be.*

> *I have the right to be treated with respect at all times. When I need a medication for pain, I should not be treated like a drug abuser.*

> *I have the right to have the pain resulting from treatments and procedures prevented, or at least minimized.*

In summary, it has been estimated that over one-million people in the United States are suffering from their cancer pain at this moment. Effective treatment for pain exists, but many people are reluctant to use it. Several conditions affect the lack of effective pain control. All health care professionals are not trained in modern pain relief methods and the caregiver, patient and others may confuse the use of drugs for pain relief with the abuse of drugs for recreation. Finally, many people have difficulty describing their pain, discussing their illness or taking drugs.

Your loved one should be as comfortable as possible with the recent advances in understanding and controlling cancer pain. Fears about addiction, sedation and other side effects are often exaggerated, and should never be a reason to stop treatment. Side effects may soon disappear or are easily treatable.

Notes from *Guidelines for Treatment of Cancer Pain,*
Texas Cancer Council, 1991

Chapter Nine

STROKE

Both a stroke, from which the victim may recover completely and Alzheimer's, which causes a gradual deterioration, may exact an overwhelming toll on the caregiver. An understanding and involved caregiver will enrich the victim's life and help dispel fear and loneliness. In this chapter and the next, you may find the tools.

"There is life and love after a stroke.
We measure days to their fullest now....
and we keep turning corners to prevent
looking back at what was."

Elaine Fantle Shimberg
Strokes: What Families Should Know

A Doctor Has a Stroke

Scheduled for minor surgery, a physician was admitted to the hospital. During the night he suffered a sudden, massive stroke and awoke so helpless that he could not speak or move. He had double vision. His shoulder felt as though it was being pulled from its socket and his head throbbed from what he thought were tiny hammers pounding continuously. Hearing intact, he listened silently as doctors and nurses discussed his slim chance of surviving the night. Locked in an immovable body, unable to speak or communicate, he did survive.

He lived in his isolation and after weeks of concentrated effort, moved one finger. The nurse noticed. Encouraged, he kept trying until he could make simple hand signals to communicate his needs: water, move, bedpan, bite, etc. He had no signal for his feelings, such as "I am afraid and lonely." He recovered, and relearned to speak and walk. Later after he had returned to an active life, he wrote an article entitled, "The Incommunicable Anonymous Order of Aphasics," offering caregivers and others a better understanding and greater insight into the lonely, confused world of the stroke victim. I offer this and other information to you.

When a loved one suffers a sudden stroke that leaves them, even temporarily, unable to navigate or make themselves understood, both they and their loved ones feel helpless. The victim of a stroke may have been thrown into an alien world, but the loved ones are in limbo. At this time, no one can explain what the future will be.

Caregivers and loved ones should keep these facts in mind:

- **Nine out of 10 stroke victims walk again.**

- **The severity of the symptoms immediately after the stroke may have little relationship to the person's ability, eventually, to return to an independent life.**

- **The residual damage to the rest of the body will be evaluated and treated while the brain has time to heal.**

What Happens When a Stroke Occurs

A clot lodges in an artery or a hemorrhage floods a part of the brain. The brain is bruised and swollen, and depending on the area, the rest of the person's body is affected. Muscles may be weak, speech and thought processes scrambled, one whole side may be paralyzed or the whole body may be immobilized. Most stroke victim's symptoms are not at either extreme, but somewhere between.

Recovery starts as the brain recovers. When the swelling in the brain goes down, the person may start to regain some speech and movement. This recovery can begin in a few days or it may take months. Recovery continues for up to two years or longer, with the greatest improvement during the first six months.

Understanding the Aftermath of a Stroke

- **Communication**

  Their amazing brain has been injured. As a result they may have one or more of the following symptoms:

  — <u>Cannot speak</u> - no matter how much they want to. They may hear the questions but cannot form the words. This is called aphasia, and they are often aware that they have it. When they can speak, the wrong word may come out. Or the throat muscles are still partially paralyzed and the words are slurred. Or their brain is still so confused that the jumble of syllables do not form words (called jargon). They usually do not know that they are speaking jargon.

  — <u>Cannot understand</u> - their brain may register a different word than the one you spoke, which makes no sense to them. You may make the meaning clearer, for instance, if you show them a glass when you ask if they want a drink.

  — <u>Have vision problems</u> - hearing is never lost, but they may have double vision. Or they may have lost a part of their visual field. If the vision is gone on the affected side, they may be unaware of that side which may affect their balance.

- **The Thought Process**

  — The ability to coordinate thoughts, remember or make a sound judgment is often affected. They may have a short attention span and will be easily distracted by sounds and movements around them.

— They often lose some control of their emotions. They cry easily - even when they are happy; may laugh inappropriately or may swear (although they never did before). Swear words, incidentally, are only meaningless words to them. Their emotional control and other abilities will improve as the brain recovers.

— A feeling of depression may be their companion during the recovery period. The depression will lighten, but may not completely leave them for some time. Remember, they are surviving in an alien world.

- **Ability To Move Around**
  — Muscle involvement may vary, from easily exhausted, weakened muscles to a paralysis of one side of the body and no muscle tone (flaccid). Even when muscles function, they may coordinate poorly. The stroke victim may not be able to pick up a book, sit down when asked to do so or start walking after standing.

  — The person may be uncomfortable. The injured brain aches and the affected muscles have prickly sensations, like a foot that is "asleep." When the stronger muscles overpower weakened ones and cause contractions, there will be some pain. If the patient tells you he hurts, his pain is real. Physical therapy should be started as soon as the acute phase is past, for flaccid muscles will gradually stiffen and contract. The exercises tone, stretch and relax muscles, so that the person may walk and use the arms and hands again.

Following a stroke, the victim may start the recovery on a general hospital floor, then be transferred to a rehabilitation unit or a long term care facility. Physical and speech therapy will be given. Your visits provide a familiar, trusted and loving presence in a world turned topsy-turvy. Remain calm, patient and optimistic. Your loved one needs a stable anchor.

Helping A Loved One Communicate

- Speak more slowly. Use familiar, ordinary words and wait for him to comprehend.

- Do not raise your voice. His hearing ability has not changed and you will give him a headache.

- Try to ask simple questions that are answered with a yes or no. Even if he cannot speak, watch the person's eyes and body movements. He may be able to write.

- Let him know when you do not understand. You are his link to the world. In general, don't correct him. Just remember that he will improve and correct himself.

- You can be honest with a stroke victim and tell him what has happened as he starts to recover. Knowledge has the ability to dispel fear. Don't be surprised if he shows his unexpressed anger. Ignored, the outbursts will soon pass.

- If he has aphasia and cannot speak, the help of a speech therapist will be needed. Therapy should be started as soon as the acute phase is over and he can get up. Ask the doctor when it will be started. The therapist will teach you how to reinforce the retraining.

Helpful Suggestions for the Caregiver:

- Comprehension is easier for him when one person talks at a time. Several people speaking is distracting. Don't over talk.

- Treat the victim of a stroke as the grown up he is, not as a child or someone who is retarded.

- The first words he will start using are nouns, followed by verbs. Use nouns when you discuss eating, dressing or toileting. He will have trouble understanding collective nouns, such as "food" or "clothing."

- Use words - bed, chair, toilet, table, clock, mouth, hand, leg, water, coffee, cigarette, soap, toothbrush, sandwich, telephone, man, money, etc. These words describe things he can see, feel or hear.

- When the person's ability to concentrate is poor, his attention span is short and he may have difficulty retaining facts. If you notice that he has become restless, starts fidgeting or looks anxious, he is being pushed. Accept his limitations and reassure him that his abilities will improve.

- Quiet music or a TV show may be enjoyable or it can be very irritating to the nervous system especially if he has a headache. Ask if he wants to listen.

- Fatigue is a constant companion. Watch for changes which indicate exhaustion - speech errors, slower thought processes, a newly acquired limp or the dragging of a foot.

Other Problems May Include:

- **Elimination**
  The loss of normal control of both voiding and bowel movements is based on the amount of injury to the brain. Control is regained as the brain heals and paralysis recedes. Constipation, while of concern, will be treated the same as with any bedfast or inactive person. The loss of control may be most upsetting to your loved one.

- **Appetite**
  A loss of appetite is a common side effect of the stroke. Depression, excess tension, altered taste sensations and

ill-fitting dentures (affected by paralysis) all may contribute to his disinterest in food. Give supplements and encourage him to drink fluids.

Tip: A person paralyzed on one side may have difficulty recognizing the amount of food remaining in his mouth or how well it has been chewed. To prevent the possibility of choking, help him to sit in a semi-upright position and turn toward his unaffected side. He will become aware of the food in his mouth.

- **Balance**

When the person walks or sits, a weakened side will pull the body in that direction. A loss of vision on the affected side allows the person to ignore that side of his body. The brain may not compensate enough to give him accurate information about the position of the leg or foot. Physical therapists will recognize these losses and will explain to you how they are helping your loved one adjust.

- **Personality**

Like a combat soldier who faces terror, brushes with death and feels trapped, the victim of a stroke may also seem different. He may be difficult and uncooperative shortly after the stroke or may be irritable, indifferent or unresponsive. Underneath all these changes the old personality is still there and intact. None of these changes will be noticed if he recovers quickly. During recovery, the person will grow more self-centered which is common with a lengthy illness. He wants meaning and order in his life. If the behavior becomes unreasonable, it isn't intentional, but is a reaction to the frustrating world he inhabits.

One authority explained that recovery from a stroke is influenced by age, physical condition, an optimistic and independent personality (pre-stroke), and how severely the brain was injured. Recovery is also influenced by the support and motivation supplied by family and friends when the person's own physical and emotional resources hit bottom.

How Best to Help Your Loved One

Develop PATIENCE. A speech therapist explains that she figuratively holds out her hands, waiting for her stroke patient to walk toward her. And he or she will move, one step at a time. The greatest recovery is achieved by the efforts of the disabled person during the time required for rehabilitation. Help them by being patient.

Remain STABLE and CONSISTENT in your approach toward your loved one. The caregiver becomes a strong, steady anchor in a loved one's strange and changing world.

Learn to GIVE CARE CORRECTLY. Ask questions, observe, and practice. Use the therapists and nurses as teachers. Your ability is a valuable asset for the recovering victim.

Provide a more STRUCTURED, CONSISTENT ENVIRONMENT with some schedules for daily activities.

Protect YOUR OWN HEALTH and ask others to help when you need them. Rest when your loved one rests.

Recovery from a Stroke

The location and size of the injury to the brain influences recovery time. Stroke victims may find speech returning in a few hours or days. Others rejoice with improvement over weeks or months. The same changes occur with paralysis of an arm or leg - the difference is that recovery is often slower. The arm and hand will recover more slowly than the leg and foot.

Many people who are left with some residual damage continue their lives as planned. They compensate for any muscle weakness by continuing the exercise program designed for them, until only a slight disability remains. Recovered, they may finish college and marry. People master the use of walkers and arm or leg braces. A continuing recovery, though slight, may extend over a number of years.

As a caregiver, remain "realistically hopeful." And work diligently with all the professional caregivers, especially during the first six months when the fastest recovery occurs. Don't lose an opportunity to strive for improvement.

Your disabled loved one must be encouraged to give his or her best efforts despite a short attention span, memory loss, mood swings and chronic fatigue. Try to recognize when you must stop pushing him and give him room to progress at his own speed. He may often feel defeated and exhausted. The person is now locked into a body which will not always do his bidding and his efforts cannot be measured by the same expectations that you have for your well-functioning body.

With the combined efforts of professional therapists, doctors, nurses and support groups, you and your loved one may be surprised and encouraged by the improvement he will make. You have helped him "turn a corner."

Chapter Ten

ALZHEIMER'S DISEASE

The caregiver of a loved one with a fatal disease lives with a sense of helplessness as she gradually loses the unique person she has known. However, she can influence the quality of the victim's life by creating a loving, permissive environment. In this chapter, many ideas and techniques are offered for stimulating remaining abilities while protecting the caregiver's sanity.

"I say 'I love you' often. In addition to being true, it gives assurance and reduces fright. When we take walks, we hold hands. That way, neither one gets lost. And that's something in life, that you don't get lost."
A quote from M.S. in <u>Aging Magazine</u> 1992

When a Loved One has Alzheimer's Disease or Other Dementia

Alzheimer's (and other dementia) can be defined as a disease of losses. From the forgetfulness of small blocks in memory to the loss of emotional control and, finally, to the loss of physical control, the disease defines and limits one's daily existence. It reverses the hierarchy of needs (Maslow) that guide our lives, starting with the loss of our highest achievements.

Jeannie Roberts, in her excellent book *Taking Care of Caregivers* describes how Alzheimer's changes and diminishes a person's world. She explains that as victims slowly lose the ability to achieve higher goals, their self-esteem begins to crumble as their skills are lost. When the ability to speak or to communicate is affected, the person is losing touch with other human beings, for they are unable to use words to express their thoughts and feelings.

As the disease progresses, they may lose the ability to understand the language of others. They will feel a sense of isolation, even when friends and family are nearby, for they no longer belong as a participant. This feeling of isolation can stimulate a perception of constant danger and may contribute to a sense of fear and paranoia. The ill person will someday be unable to protect and care for himself without a caregiver's help.

At this time, 1995, the process cannot be stopped or reversed, but may be slowed. As the caregiver, you should help your loved one function at his most capable level for as long as possible. Your care will make a difference in his life. Physical exercise, stimulation of the mind and the senses plus the use of available drugs, all help slow the gradual loss of the familiar person you love.

The disease can be loosely divided into three stages - early, middle and late. A diagnosis is difficult in the early stages, for it is easy to deny the changes, justify the symptoms and delay seeking medical advice. Symptoms begin with forgetfulness and a memory loss for names, day-to-day recall, the day of the month and where items were placed. Aware of this loss, the person becomes anxious and rude at times.

As the forgetfulness increases, and he cannot recall recent events, he may feel confused. He may become agitated, weep, be angry or at times, stubborn. He may have rapid mood swings. These reactions may last for a short time until his usual pleasant disposition returns. How difficult and how frustrating it must be for him to try to remain independent!

The Caregiver's Contributions

The diagnosis of Alzheimer's, like cancer or Aids, is often as difficult for the caregiver to accept as the person who is ill. It is understandable that each may feel overwhelmed and deny the truth. When you, as the caregiver, accept that you are powerless to stop the progress of the disease, a sense of guilt may linger. You understand intellectually, but emotionally still feel responsible.

Jeannie Roberts reminds the caregiver that you have much to offer. You should:

- Take time to grieve together, mend fences and express how much you love each other, for later your loved one might not understand or appreciate your words.

- Start to make plans so the ill person may continue to live independently for as long as possible.

- Consider sources for respite care and other types of needed assistance as the illness progresses. Take time to evaluate the nursing homes in your area. Many have special Alzheimer's wings.

- Encourage your loved one to put his affairs in order while still capable of decision making. He should make a living will, regular will or trust and might discuss any preferences for the funeral.

Over the years, as your loved one becomes more dependent, the confinement of daily caregiving can overwhelm and exhaust you. Without outside help, the strongest caregiver will eventually break down. Help is available in the community and a caregiver should learn when and how to use these resources:

Adult day care	Alternative housing
Meals-on-Wheels	Family support groups
Visiting nurses	Family violence programs
Respite care	Alcohol/drug abuse programs
Transportation	Nursing homes
Homemaker services	Hospice care
Medical and legal assistance	Financial assistance

Call the local chapter of the Alzheimer's Disease and Related Disorders Association for up-to-date information and an invitation to attend the support group. You may find information from the county Department on Aging, the Public Health Nursing department and the telephone yellow pages. Find an advocate if you need any help to cut the red tape of government agencies.

You must take care of yourself. Never attempt to "go it alone." Friends and relatives may say, "Call me if I can help", and mean it. Build a network of substitute caregivers who will do specific things on a regular basis. Do not isolate yourself with daily responsibilities or try to cope with your loneliness alone. You are very valuable to your loved one and you have a responsibility to take care of yourself.

Remember to take each day as it comes. The past is over and need not be relived. Enjoy the shared moments today, for the future is uncertain. Worrying about tomorrow only makes today more stressful.

Create a Comfortable Home Environment

When you step into a home, you notice the physical surroundings and sense the emotional field that has been created. Some homes seem warm and comfortable while others are cold and empty. You can change the home you share with a loved one (with Alzheimer's) to make life easier for both of you. A warm, permissive home can change your loved one's attitude and reactions. It is a small sacrifice for you. Keep in mind that his behavior is defensive and fearful, for he is defending himself from something he does not understand. He becomes agitated because he is confused about the world around him. You can create a calm, safe environment.

Start with physical changes:

- Place a lock or hook either up high or down low on outside doors. If the person tends to wander, add a simple doorknob alarm that beeps when the knob is turned. These are battery operated devices which fasten on the knob, and are found in children's toy outlets or electronic stores.

- Try to use bright, solid colors, contrasted where possible, so the person can find his place at the kitchen table, locate a favorite lounge chair and go to his bed. A favorite Afghan, pillow, brightly colored plate or coffee mug may remind him where to sit. Vivid patterns and stripes may overstimulate him and brightly flowered material may appear real.

- Loud noises, a blaring television or radio, people yelling or a phone that continues to ring may make him fearful and agitated. Keep the noise level lower and consider using a chime on the phone.

- Pick up throw rugs and whatnots to clear pathways throughout the house. Be alert for sharp edges and trailing electric cords.

- As the disease progresses, remove most of the clothes from his closet, so he can decide more easily what to wear. Or lay an outfit of clothes out for the next day.

- Purchase the plastic door restraints used for children (found in toy or hardware stores). Put dangerous substances or valuable objects in drawers or cabinets, fasten and explain "that drawer does not work."

- Paint the inside of drawers white and use large drawer or door pulls. Keep the rooms well lighted during the day if he has visual changes, such as decreased depth perception, blurred vision or a poor ability to distinguish contrasts. Use several lamps around the room to offer a lower, more diffused light at night so glare and shadows are reduced. Shadows may appear to be dark holes to him. Do not place a light directly over the head of the bed.

- The person may be unable to find the bathroom, and needs a picture of a toilet on the door. Place a ribbon, picture of a bed or the person's name on a bedroom door for his benefit.

- Consider household products that may be toxic. The person may consider mouthwash a pleasant mint drink.

- Install safety bars in the bathroom, handrails where needed and add a foam insert to elevate the toilet seat.

Create a Comfortable Emotional Environment

One experienced caregiver explained that you should become bilingual and speak "Alzheimer's," a largely nonverbal body language. Create a relaxed environment that offers easy choices and simple tasks with little risk of failure. The tasks should not provoke fear or a stubborn refusal when his self-esteem is threatened. Encourage him to do what he can do well for himself or with a little help. You learn to understand what he is feeling, not what he says.

The person with Alzheimer's absorbs others' emotions. If you are angry, he will react angrily, and, without understanding why, will continue to feel angry. When you are happy, he will have the same emotional response. You must listen carefully to the comments. When a man asked, "Where will I sleep tonight?" he wanted to find his room where he felt safe. Put your arms around him to help him feel safe.

Suggestions to help prevent a feeling of anxiety:

- Wait until it is time to leave the house to announce your plans if he begins to worry when told earlier.

- Write your answer on a piece of paper if the patient repeatedly asks the same question. He can look at the answer.

- Change the TV to another program if one seems to make him restless and anxious. He may no longer understand a serious program but may enjoy Sesame Street.

Tips for Caregiving During the Stages of Illness
The Early Stages - (First stage - 2-4 years)

Physical Exercise

Continue the activities your loved one enjoys (swimming, dancing, bike riding, playing ball)

Take walks, even short walks, for the person needs to walk to reduce their agitation.

If he sits most of the time, encourage stretching exercises. Have him lift both arms and legs, lean and twist the body and squeeze a rubber ball for hand and finger exercises.

Note: Avoid physical restraints which will add to his confusion.

Communication

This may be the last time to reminisce, share photo albums and remember happy occasions. You may travel together and enjoy visits with the special people in your loved one's life. Use this last opportunity to enrich his life and to provide happy memories of carefree times together.

Mental Stimulation During the Early and Middle Stages

You must realize that as your loved one's brain changes, he or she may experience unexpected losses. The losses may not have a pattern. One day the person may be functioning fairly well and the next day a simple task is impossible. Be observant. If you fail to recognize and to accept the loss, insisting that he can do the task, he will be frustrated and the symptoms will become worse. When he loses the ability to continue his hobbies: sports, cards, puzzles, reading etc., try to keep the brain more alert by:

- Reading simple stories, poetry, Bible stories, newspapers.

- Including your loved one in group conversations.

- Placing pictures of family, friends and of himself near him. Choose older pictures rather than recent ones.

- Keeping a clock in the room and making a large weekly calender.

Note: Some people with dementia enjoy rearranging furniture in a doll house or tinkering with a clock or appliances which they can take apart. Working in the yard or gardening may keep them occupied. One company, Geriatric Resources, offers a long apron with large pockets, a zipper, buttons etc. on the front.

During the Middle Stages - (Second stage - 2 to 10 years)

Visual Stimulation

During these stages the person may have a short attention span. Think of things that may catch his attention, such as:

- Add colorful pictures in the room. Put large, brightly-colored labels on the door to identify each room. Make or buy a colorful mobile and place in the room or near a chair. Put a pot of colorful flowers in the room or plant some outside.

- Provide coloring books and crayons. Sometimes he may use artwork to communicate when he can no longer find the words.

- Give him a set of colorful building blocks. Find a set of coordination blocks (different shapes that fit in similar holes).

- Encourage him to help with small tasks such as making a bed, washing dishes, etc.

Hearing /Sound Stimulation

- Play music that your loved one enjoyed when he was young. Encourage him to keep time to the music.

- Make or buy simple rhythm instruments such as children's plastic ones. Use an empty oatmeal box for a drum. Encourage him to play along with a familiar record. Play soft, soothing music at bedtime.

- Ask friends to tape messages. Talk about things they did together in years past and sing songs they both enjoyed.

- Speak softly unless the person is hard of hearing. Do NOT speak harshly.

- Have a house pet (cat, dog or even a bird) as a companion.

General Tips for Caregiving with Alzheimer's

- Communicate in a clear, direct manner. Use short sentences and don't give the person choices.

- If he is confused, place the mattress and box springs on the floor for safety. Use night lights.

- Buy sturdy shoes with soles that will not slip.

- Use his forgetfulness when he refuses to do something. Wait a few minutes and ask again.

- Use disposable briefs if incontinence is a problem.

- Offer something to drink every few hours for he may forget to drink fluids.

- Serve several small meals during the day. Serve meals in the same place and about the same time each day. When choices make him confused, serve one food item at a time. Moisten the food by adding broth, gravy or sauces.

- Meals with varied and colorful food may be enjoyable after some other senses are gone. Serve precut or bite-size food in casseroles and stews (shred meat instead of grinding), and try not to serve baby food. Serve ice cream and flavorful drinks.

- Try giving some carbohydrates, such as fruit or sweets at bedtime in place of a sleeping pill.

- Your loved one's tastes may change. If he adds an excessive amount of salt or sugar to the food, remove the seasonings from the table.

- Check hearing aid batteries weekly. Be sure glasses are worn and check that the lens are clean and not scratched.

- Sometimes he may become frightened by something you cannot see. Remove a picture or whatever seems frightening if you can.

- Pleasant odors (potpourri for one) and familiar odors such as bread baking, may be soothing to him.

- Your loved one will feel comforted by a hug, a pat or holding hands. When he no longer responds to sights or voices, he will be soothed when lovingly touched.

- A back rub and gentle massage will relax his tired muscles.

- Stimulate the sense of touch with fluffy blankets, furry toys, cool water, a stiff brush, etc.

- Have the person wear an identification bracelet. Hide the car keys when he is no longer able to drive.

- Maintain eye contact, listen attentively and avoid confrontations. Always call him by name.

Care During The Later Stages - (Terminal stage - 1-3 years)

Changes Due to Brain Degeneration

Your loved one may be confused and often will not understand what is being discussed. Use short sentences and wait to see if he understands. If he seems agitated use a soothing, calm voice, fix a cup of warm tea or coffee (caffeine-free), and go for a short walk together.

Start asking questions, such as, "Did something scare you?" "Do you need to use the bathroom?" "Are you worried?" and ask him, "Do you need a hug?"

A person's skills slowly disappear with Alzheimer's, although not all skills are affected equally. The ability to understand what is being said may outlast the ability to speak. So use gestures when you talk to demonstrate what you are saying. Also try breaking everyday tasks into easy steps and tell him each step. "Eat your food" becomes "Take a bite of your meat loaf." Or if you ask him to step into the tub, and he just stands there, say "Pick up your foot."

When the person can no longer speak, watch the familiar body language, for it is his only method of communication. Even if he can speak, the words may not be what he means. Since you can read his body language as easily as he reads yours, you may notice that he is very relieved when you understand his needs.

After the person is non-responsive and becomes bedfast, he will hear your words and feel your touch. So talk softly, pray, read and tell him that you care. Rub the neck and shoulders, hold his hand and pat him often. These signs of affection are very comforting in a silent, isolated world.

The Caregiver's Self Protection

Despite the pain, you must find ways to cope with your grief and sadness as you gradually lose the person you knew. You may often feel powerless and frustrated, and unexpectedly, may feel hostile for a brief time. Caregiving is confining. Jeannie Roberts explains that you will recognize how the daily stresses have affected your behavior when you:

- Are always in a hurry and often late.

- Have trouble concentrating, planning your day, finishing one job.

- Are often irritable, find fault, anger easily, and yell or cry.

- Have a poor appetite, feel tired but have difficulty sleeping.

- Feel depressed and seem to have mood swings.

When you no longer see yourself as the humorous, loving, forgiving person you are and note that your zest for life has been replaced by a sense of frustration and loneliness, you must take care of yourself. You must guard against the escapes of overeating, chain smoking or excess spending.

To unwind and protect your health, find a plan of action that works for you. Use these stress-managing techniques:

- Eat good meals and limit your use of caffeine, salt or alcohol. Drink plenty of water, juices and beverages to keep the body's fluids and chemicals balanced.

- Let your body have an adequate amount of undisturbed rest. Nerves need to "unwind" - so find someone to replace you for a few hours while you sleep.

- Practice taking deep breaths to get more oxygen in your body, and then stretch your muscles.
    - Lie in bed on your side and stretch your hand over your head as high as you can reach. At the same time point your toe and try to stretch the foot downward. (Stretch like a cat.) Hold rigidly for a few moments, then suddenly relax. Turn to the other side and repeat.
    - Lie comfortably in bed and start relaxing, from the head, neck, face and shoulders down to your toes. Go slowly and once relaxed, lie quietly for 15 minutes.
    - Go outside every day together and walk, walk, walk.

- Never try to carry the total responsibility alone. Visit with someone who will not be shocked, not give advice or repeat your unguarded comments - then feel free to unload.

- Find something to punch if anger and frustration builds up. Try a pillow or fill a long sock with other socks and pound on a chair, bed or car fender. Gain a healthy release.

Note: Suggestions to help keep you sane:
Keep in touch with friends. Take others' advice and criticism with a grain of salt.

Live one day at a time. Enjoy each new morning.

Repeat the serenity prayer and accept the limits of what you can accomplish.

Take a moment to consider your own life. Remind yourself that you are valuable - a person worth knowing.

The Danger of Abuse

I would be remiss if I did not discuss the abuse that can develop, both unconsciously and consciously. All family relationships are not stable, sharing or loving. The caregiver may remember harsh words with unfair treatment, or being ignored, excluded or abused. The person with Alzheimer's may not feel close to his caregiver. Both people may try to wipe out and forgive the past. The sick person, because of the illness, has a poor ability to cope with anger, exhaustion, frustration and continued losses. His unreasonable actions increase the stress on the most patient caregiver, which may result in abuse. If a caregiver ever attempts to "get even," the cycle of abuse continues. The ill person is really very helpless.

How to Prevent Ever Becoming Abusive

- **Get away from the situation.**
  Take a breather.
  Physical abuse is never, never justified. A caregiver for someone with dementia may find themselves on the verge of violence at times. The ill loved one may become combative (out of fear) or angry and aggressive as the brain deteriorates. Understanding the actions does not make it less frustrating for you, the caregiver.

- **Seek professional help.**
  When you realize you are dangerously close to lashing out (or have been abusive), talk with a counselor, nurse, doctor, minister or a support group leader. Do it now. (Remember, many counselors in agencies work on sliding scale fees.) If you feel that you are unable to cope, start making plans for another place for the ill person to live.

- **Admit your loved one to a nursing home.**
  There are two reasons to consider a nursing home:
  — Every caregiver has limitations. Eventually, the ill person may be so impaired that everyone in the house is being damaged by the constant stress.
  — In a nursing home, as many as five to eight staff members will provide the daily care that you have been giving at home. The staff in a capably-staffed, well-run nursing home have been trained to handle difficult behaviors.

In Summary -

Over one million people have a dementing illness today. If each illness affects three people, around four million people are trying to cope with these disabling conditions. Over half the caregivers are spouses and another third are the children who may have families of their own. The questions they ask include, "When should we consider admitting him or her to a nursing home?" and "Once diagnosed, how long does my loved one have to live?"

During a small study, fourteen Alzheimer's patients were monitored and evaluated every six months for a two-year period. The study showed that the disease progresses at a fairly stable rate. It was unusual if some changes were not noted from one six-month check to the next. Patients were at various levels of impairment when the study began. During the next two years, twelve of the fourteen patients were admitted to a nursing home. The three conditions, together, which were the deciding factors for admission were:

- Incontinence, a loss of control of kidney and/or bowel function.

- Unable to speak coherently, to make themselves understood, and the ability to recognize family members.

- Needed assistance with all basic daily grooming.

The final decision to admit a loved one to a nursing home is usually a difficult one, as families struggle to do what is best for the person who is ill. A center which provides capable, loving care will free the exhausted caregivers to enjoy visits, provide stimulation and offer comfort.

Note: The life expectancy from the onset of Alzheimer's is roughly estimated from five to ten years, although the progressive changes vary from one individual to another.

Chapter Eleven

CHRONIC CONDITIONS THAT INFLUENCE CAREGIVING

Your loved one may have other chronic conditions. These may range from mildly to progressively debilitating, and while not the primary disability, may require your attention, time and assistance. Three very different conditions which require attention are emphysema, paralysis and personality problems.

Chronic Obstructive Lung Disease (Emphysema and Others)

A disabled loved one may have his life complicated by a shortness of breath due to emphysema or another chronic obstructive lung disease (COPD.) Environmental pollution, as well as heavy cigarette smoking influences the higher incidence of COPD today. You can help the person live much more comfortably when you follow the doctor's suggestions when preparing meals, observe and evaluate his abdominal breathing and share exercise times.

You should understand what has happened to the lungs with emphysema. Inside the lung, the fragile walls of several tiny air sacks have broken, forming a small pocket. When enough of these pockets exist, they will hold some stagnant air, and eventually some secretions, preventing fresh air (oxygen) from filling the pocket. During exertion, the person becomes short of breath as he runs short of available oxygen. By learning to "belly breathe," the diaphragm works more effectively. He will use the abdominal muscles to help empty and refill the lungs with oxygen, which will help his shortness of breath.

Controlled Diaphramatic Breathing (Belly Breathing) Technique

This is a learned type of breathing, which initially seems odd, but assures the maximum intake of oxygen with the greatest removal of carbon dioxide. It helps prevent physical exhaustion and will lighten feelings of depression. You, the caregiver, should practice the "belly breathing" technique, so you will be able to observe and correct your loved one. Remind him to belly breathe as he lifts, reaches or sits up before getting out of bed. The technique is easily learned and becomes second nature with practice:

- With body erect and shoulders relaxed, inhale through the nose with the mouth shut. The upper chest should not rise as air is pulled in slowly and smoothly.

- Make the upper abdomen slowly balloon outward while inhaling. This helps lower the diaphragm and pulls more air into the lungs. Hold the breath for a few seconds before exhaling.

- Exhale slowly by opening and pursing the lips to form a small 0 and blowing. Using this technique, he helps hold the breathing passages open longer, allowing more waste carbon dioxide to be eliminated. Exhaling should take twice as long as inhaling.

Note: As one starts to exhale, the upper abdomen will sink back normally, and not from an effort to squeeze. When he has finished exhaling, however, the abdominal muscles should be used to squeeze the last waste air from the lungs.

If someone with COPD becomes short of breath, help him relax.

Excitement makes breathing more difficult. Remind him to try to deflate the lungs to get rid of excess stale air. To do this he should:
Purse his lips as he exhales and use both hands to push the upper abdomen inward and upward. He will inhale, then repeat this way of exhaling several times.

Other Suggestions to Help a Person with COPD

- Go walking together. Start slowly, walking a little farther each time. Don't let him become exhausted. Stop often to rest and chat.

- Make a work or hobby area on a table large enough to hold all work materials. Find a comfortable chair of the right height for the table. The person can save energy by working slowly and smoothly, using both hands, working from left to right instead of back and forth and alternating light and heavy tasks.

- Plan several small meals each day with a very light evening meal. Salt should be omitted. Remind the person to take small bites and chew with their mouth closed. This prevents swallowing air and a distended stomach which makes breathing more difficult.

- Personal care will be easier if a chair or stool is placed in the tub, a hand-held sprayer is used and grab bars are installed. Shoes and clothing should be easy to slip on.

- Control the environment with an evaporation humidifier in dry climates and fans or air conditioning in summer. Room humidity should be kept at 30-50%. Air-warming masks and warm clothes offer protection in winter. Keep the home free of smoke, aerosol sprays, fumes and heavy dust.

- The person should stay away from anyone with an upper respiratory infection. Calm a stressful situation and suggest a nap if he does not sleep well.

- Contact the doctor if his mucous production increases, thickens, changes color or contains blood. Observe his ankles for swelling and listen for increased breathlessness. If your loved one has not had flu or pneumonia shots as a preventative measure, inform the doctor.

From Activities of Daily Living for Patients with COPD
Glasrock Home Health Care booklet

Coping with a Permanent Disability

Your caregiving may begin shortly after your loved one is permanently disabled or years later. He may still be struggling to master the use of a wheelchair or may have grown comfortable with his limitations. This disability may be secondary to his major debilitating condition, but he needs your help to maintain his independence and your emotional support as he copes with a future forever changed.

The Response to Loss

Your loved one has sustained a sudden injury so severe that it produces a permanent loss, such as a spinal cord injury, and you share his shock and numbness. Another person with a chronic disease which causes intermittent losses, such as multiple sclerosis, allows his loved ones the time to adjust. Each person's loss may be equally as great, the pain and frustration as real, but the time factor makes the difference.

Initially, with a sudden traumatic loss, the protective shock prevents anxiety, until the injured person begins to understand the reality of his condition. During the period of denial which follows, he may become angry with you or blame someone else for the disability. But he cannot ignore what has happened for long and will give up his denial - protective as it has been.

He may decide that with determination, hard work, the right treatments and enough time, he will recover and so he rejects activities designed to help him function with his disability. Time passes while he struggles until he slowly accepts that the loss is permanent. The person's life has changed and he will grieve for the important things that are lost. His pride and self-esteem are affected and he may feel of little value. He may fleetingly entertain thoughts of suicide. His moods may swing from angry and hostile to withdrawn and seemingly resigned. Finally, he will "rope off" areas that no one else may trespass, and feel that it is his life, his loss, his space. In time, when the mourning and pain ease, the doors he has closed will open.

The person with a chronic, progressive condition may become as equally disabled, but the losses "come in small bites." He must face the same losses as he struggles with the hope for improvement undermined by anxiety when the condition worsens. The painful steps toward acceptance are the same.

You, as caregiver, often have time to accept the loss and to mourn for plans which must be abandoned while the disabled one is still traveling his lonely road. You offer your support and understanding, but cannot save him from the painful process of adjustment. Surviving the ordeal may provide the courage for him to rebuild his future using the abilities he has left. With each success, his self-esteem grows as well as his determination to go on. The disability has been recognized and accepted. Finally, your loved one's ability to function more independently puts everything in perspective.

It has taken time for your loved one to realize that he is a person aside from the disability. He will see beyond and around it. This acceptance and understanding completes the adjustment to his loss for he may again become frustrated, angry or sad, which are normal emotions, but he will continue with his plans.

Ways To Help a Paralyzed or Progressively Disabled Loved One

- Be an asset, not a hindrance. Make short, daily hospital visits and ask the nurse to explain any changes in his condition.

- Remain calm if he is angry. Remind him how important he is in your life. Be patient.

- Be consistent and supportive. Ask the therapists to define the limits of the support that is needed.

- Do not perform tasks for him that he is capable of doing. It robs him of a pride in hard-earned achievements.

- Ask the nurses to teach you how to give the care needed.

- Do not be overprotective. Appreciate his new independence and stop telling him what to do.

Note: This description of the mourning and acceptance process has been included to help you understand the stages of adjustment. You should recognize and appreciate the progress the person has made. He or she may seem angry or depressed for a long time and should move forward to an acceptance of the condition. However, we all cope on our own timetable, and you must give him the time he needs to struggle through his pain.

The Caregiver's Contribution

Keep in mind that you are not accountable for your loved one's adjustment. The process must take place inside his head, as he considers the strengths he has left and tests to see how much he can accomplish. As much as you want to, you cannot either force acceptance or give him a new sense of self worth. His self-image has changed and he will mourn the loss of the person he knew. With the realization that life cannot continue as before, he will wonder how his relationships with family and friends have changed, if he will be rejected or if someone will try to control his future. He feels vulnerable and can be influenced at this time by others' expectations.

You help when you are honest and consistent and:

- See him as the same person he was before the disability.

- Accept the new limitations and help him evaluate the remaining abilities.

- Give him the freedom and space to work through the anger and frustration.

- Maintain a stable home with your humor and love.

- Share his concerns, but do not express your doubts and fears.

- Remember that a person's life belongs to him and his personal successes are important to him.

Comment: If the disabled person has been very unhappy with his life, he might view his new dependence as acceptable. He would welcome the care and concern of the hospital staff and enjoy the continuing sympathy and thoughtfulness of others. If his dependency also meets the needs of a family member or friend, this person might encourage his helplessness and cooperate. For instance, the disabled person who insists on care months after he or she is quite able to manage alone, and the relative who encourages the long-term dependency, are each meeting their own needs. The disabled loved one's loss has become important to both of them.

This type of co-dependent relationship is the exception. The family members and the disabled loved one's goal must be the same - that he achieve as much independence as possible.

Coping with a Difficult Person

Your disabled person may have a reason to be upset or angry. But if disagreements do not get resolved and are carried over from day to day, the house may seem too small to find relief from the turmoil. Whatever the cause - anger over the disabling condition, an ongoing feud, painful past memories, abuse of drugs or alcohol, or personality quirks - day to day bickering can become unbearable. You are living with a difficult person. Have you become difficult too?

When discussions become duels and silences stop further communication, you both need a "breather." You need time and space to allow emotions to cool and conflicts to shrink to reasonable proportions. The issues are seldom as simple as they seem. The real problem may be hidden under angry words and irritating actions. The person who responds with strong emotions fails to search for the underlying cause of such anger. Those who are closely associated have learned which "buttons to push" to get a response.

One caregiver knew she must find help when she began to resent the visitors who always complimented her disabled husband's efforts, but ignored her hard work. She performed all the daily chores, cared for their children and met his needs. She was ashamed of her petty attitude and that she resented her courageous husband. Because of her exhaustion, she grew angry. The situation changed when she located a capable part-time caregiver, asked her teenage sons to be responsible for part of the household chores and discussed the situation with a counselor.

Problems will not miraculously disappear, but one quickly recognizes that strong emotions are exhausting and destroy a sense of peace and harmony. Life is no longer pleasant as conflicts become unwanted burdens. You and your loved one may be motivated to improve your relationship when given the time to regain a more balanced perspective. During a calm discussion, you may be able to listen to each other's viewpoint, search for acceptable solutions and become more forgiving.

Plans for a short respite from caregiving must include competent replacement care for your loved one. Volunteer caregivers may not be available or remain long if they are. A home health agency staff member can provide short-term care on short notice. Released from daily confinement you have the privacy to regain some objectivity. The more serious differences may be difficult to resolve. A trained, impartial counselor will help you identify your choices and possible solutions. To continue in a stressful situation, without changing it, only creates more turmoil. Agencies, such as Family Service, have experienced counselors, and their fee is based on a sliding-scale rate calculated on one's income.

You are not alone if you wonder where you may find competent help. Employing a full-time caregiver will give you the freedom to pursue your interests, but the expense may be prohibitive. Consider hiring a part-time caregiver to give specific care.

Another possibility is the use of a day care center. You might make arrangements for your loved one to visit the center. Investigate the type of daily activities offered, type of food served and space provided for naps. If the person is able to walk, even with help, or is wheelchair bound, investigate the local transportation systems which offer door-to-door rides for disabled. The transportation and the center visit, for a few hours or a full day, are inexpensive.

You may recruit family members, willing neighbors and old friends to form a respite network. When asked, they may agree to give a few hours of relief care each week. The total hours may offer you and your loved one freedom from a daily routine. Be alert for an experienced caregiver who may agree to barter a few hours time for a service you can trade (sewing, homemade bread, for example.)

As you prepare to discuss the problems which have created the turmoil, consider:

- **The only person you can change or control is you.** Time and effort is often wasted trying to change the other person.

- **Strive for calmness and reason.**
  Patience and a willingness to listen often open channels for discussion. When people can agree, they may find solutions.

- **Forgiveness is a great healer.**
  The bitterness from past mistreatment with seemingly unforgivable actions becomes a heavy burden to keep alive each day. You may forgive another person for your own sake, in order to wipe out your anger and pain. It is difficult to feel comfortable with yourself, to share joy or trust others, when you remain furious. You can still protect yourself from being mistreated again.

- **A loved one's controlling weaknesses or neurotic personality need to be evaluated objectively.**
  You may be too intimately involved and have lost the ability to influence the situation. An impartial, professional (psychologist, social worker or minister) may offer valuable help to both of you.

Comment: I assume that you will read this book because you want to be a more capable caregiver. As you discuss a problem situation, your own actions cannot be ignored. Consider these questions:

- Are you careless about personal hygiene? Is your body odor offensive and/or your breath foul? Do you contaminate the air with heavy cigarette smoke?

- Do you give care resentfully? Are you slow to help? Do you complain and blame others?

- Do you try to control the disabled person and not ask his opinions or accept his wishes?

- Do you enjoy a "good fight" and try to have the last word?

- Have you used your role as constant caregiver as a reason to indulge in overeating, excessive drinking or gambling?

- How much responsibility must you take for these problems and how willing are you to correct them?

How to Cope with Two Difficult Problems

Alcohol or Drug Abuse

You, as the caregiver, cannot ignore a loved one's substance abuse. You need to find ways to cope with your disappointment and frustration. The addicted person must wage the battle to free himself. You must concentrate on saving your own sanity.

A doctor specializing in rehabilitative medicine was asked how she copes with patients who have a drug or drinking problem. She explains at the beginning of their association that she will give her best efforts toward their recovery and expects the same from them. She warns against the use of "crutches" such as alcohol or drugs. If any patient comes to therapy under the influence of a substance, she gives one warning. She reminds the patient that the effort needed for recovery is hard enough, and that if he does not seek help and continues the abuse, she will ask him to find another doctor.

An addicted person needs the support of recovering addicts. One alcoholic described his feelings during his time of addiction:

"I saw myself on a straight toboggan slide to skid row - with no way to get off. I hated myself for being the way I was, and I felt over and over, day after week after month after year, that I was in a steel box running round and round on a treadmill that went faster and faster - with no way out. The most terrible part of this experience was that I was going through it entirely alone. I couldn't bring myself to talk about it, even with my wife. She thought I didn't care and drank because I enjoyed it. I cared more than I could say."

He explained that when an alcoholic attends an A.A. meeting, he or she has a "fantastic sense of relief." They can talk to someone who understands and cares. The person can open up about his secret fears and humiliations, and, with other members' support, regain a measure of confidence that he, too, can remain sober one day at a time.

The abuser must travel his own road to recovery. Loved ones who have adjusted their lives to "picking up the pieces" will wonder how they can help. They need answers to questions, such as:

"How much responsibility can the recovering person accept?"

"Are other A.A. members the only people they need?"

"Who offers the family support if their loved one slips?"

Alanon, the auxiliary organization to A.A., offers the same kind of help to family members. During the meetings, they will find answers to their questions, although members do not give advice, and will soon realize how they can change and make adjustments as the addict recovers. A caregiver and other family members can find help and support at an Alanon meeting before a loved one is ready to end his addiction.

Coping with the Neurotic Person

Dr. Albert Ellis in his book, *How to Live with a Neurotic* describes a neurotic person as:

"One who has feelings of worthlessness and inadequacy because he is supersensitive and magnifies his faults. He is fearful that others will not approve of him, fears making a mistake and thus failing in everyone's eyes. He views the world as unfair.

Instead of facing the facts of life, the person tends to evade issues, blame others, rationalize and create a more rosy world. Because he feels insecure, he may adopt a rigid set of rules for himself. And because he keeps muscles and nervous system in a state of tension, he will tend to have physical ailments.

The neurotic person has a great desire to receive love, but because of the concern with problems, has a smaller capacity to give love. If he compensates well enough, he may be outwardly content, but may feel intensely depressed at times. If alcohol or drugs are used to try to escape reality, these "crutches" boomerang because his confidence is not increased."

When loved ones and others realize how constantly the person struggles to cope, it becomes easier to understand how helpless and lonely he feels. He recognizes that he is considered a misfit, but protects his vulnerability, and is not easily changed."

Dr. Ellis offers these guidelines for caregivers and loved ones:

- Don't behave too neurotically yourself. Remain calm, patient and reasonable.

- Accept that a neurotic person may act both normal and at times, rather peculiarly.

- Don't take the behavior personally, for he or she will treat others as they treat themselves.

- Love him - in a cautious, toned-down way and keep your perspective. He can give just so much because of his self protection.

- Give her warmth and support, even when she seems to go out of the way to bring on disapproval. She can more easily accept and forgive herself if you accept her, unconditionally, despite her actions.

- Adopt an attitude of "firm kindness," acting nicely but setting definite limits as to how he may impose on you - and firmly stick to those limits.

- Keep a rational, realistic philosophy about life.

- Finally, do something to relieve a neurotic loved one's feelings of guilt. Discuss his or her actions in a lenient, non-threatening way. Encourage him to do what he considers to be right.

In summary, do not criticize, for criticism is taken too seriously. **Critical words rarely move people to constructive action.** The answer is love. Out of love for someone, a person will move in a different direction. If he feels that you care and can see things from his viewpoint, he will feel that he has a true helper and a better chance to overcome fears.

Living with a difficult person is never easy. Since you only have the power to change yourself, try not to let emotions rule the situation. Consider the choices available to you. Forgive the other person for your sake. The more calm, reasonable and compassionate you feel, the better decisions you will make in any situation. Your wise choices may influence your angry, fearful loved one more than any loud argument.

Give yourself a respite. A kind, dependable relief caregiver is worth the search and the cost. The free time will give the two of you the space and relief to regain a sense of humor. It is the quality of daily life for both of you that counts. Difficult people yearn for a peaceful, fulfilled life. They do not always know how to achieve it.

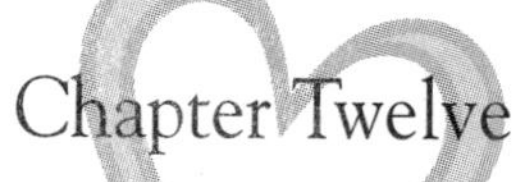

Chapter Twelve

EMERGENCIES AND THE HOSPITAL STAY

911 has become our emergency lifeline for help. Caregivers should be able to perform CPR competently and support one's life until help arrives. Later, as a hospital visitor, the caregiver should feel comfortable. This chapter discusses the unwritten rules of the hospital and how to resolve any concerns you may have.

Emergency Situation - 911 Call

Every caregiver of a chronically ill loved one should be prepared to call for help in an emergency. Review the following steps:

If the person appears unresponsive or unconscious, shake his shoulder. If no response, check if he is breathing.

Call 911 or the local emergency number if there is no 911 in the area. Give the operator the following information:

STATE: I HAVE A MEDICAL EMERGENCY.
GIVE: NAME, PHONE NUMBER, ADDRESS
STATE BRIEFLY WHAT HAS HAPPENED.
STATE IF PERSON IS BREATHING OR NOT BREATHING.

Comment: In larger cities, your name and address are flashed on the screen. When a cellular phone is used, however, no information is provided. If you live in a rural area, give directions to your home.

The emergency operator (dispatcher) is trained to offer assistance, and will give you instructions. Stay calm and talk to the operator. The operator will notify the fire and police department as you talk.

Before help arrives, unlock the entrance door. Check that a pathway is cleared and give your loved one a quick check. Here's what to do if the person:

- **Has a poor exchange of air.**
If you hear snoring, rattling or rasping sounds (he or she appears unconscious), lift the point of the chin upward, turn the head to the side or reach in and clean out the mouth. Pull the tongue forward. Do NOT turn or tilt the head if you suspect a neck injury.

If the person seems to be having a convulsion, roll him onto his side, but keep your hand out of the mouth. Do not restrain him.

- **Is bleeding from cuts or tears.**
Check for bleeding and if seen, grab a clean cloth (washcloth), cover the cut and press firmly directly over the cut. Look for a stream of spurting blood and stop it first.

- **Feels cold and has a gray look.**
The trauma from an accident, loss of blood or a serious illness can put the body in shock. Cover him with a blanket, coat or whatever is handy. Elevate his feet on pillows (unless you suspect an injury).

Keep talking to a loved one, even if you believe he is unconscious. If semi-conscious or having had a stroke, he may hear your words and be reassured. Reassure him that help is on the way.

When help arrives, answer questions and step out of the way. Try to relax. Ride in the EMS vehicle or with a friend if you are too upset to drive.

Note: Pharmacies, funeral homes and others give stickers with emergency numbers to be placed on the phone. Plan how you will respond in an emergency. You may save valuable minutes. Take a course in CPR and practice until you can perform a smooth, efficient technique. Remember, if your performance is not perfect under stress - <u>some CPR is better than no CPR</u>.

The Hospital Stay

Your disabled loved one has been admitted to the hospital. If you wish to be an asset to the patient, feel at ease and cope with any problems that might arise, you should know the written and unwritten rules of the hospital.

Hospital facilities and procedures are designed to meet the needs of the patients. Their visitors wait in uncomfortable chairs, eat too much junk food from vending machines and survive with a few hours of interrupted sleep. You are anxious, tousled, uncomfortable and feel you are in the way. You may find it difficult to relinquish the protective caregiver role to the doctor and nurses.

It is time to take care of you. You need to go home, take a warm bath and sleep in your own bed. If you are too worried to fall asleep or are awake during the night, call the hospital and ask for an updated report. Busy nurses will take a minute to reassure an anxious loved one.

The Unwritten Rules of the Hospital

On admission, the patient and family members receive a brochure listing the policies (rules) of the hospital. You will feel more comfortable when you understand the unwritten rules also. These include:

- **Visiting a patient.**

  Hospital patients need extra rest. The commotion caused by visitors, combined with unfamiliar hospital sounds, often prevents this. Some hospitals have open visiting hours and patients may be visited anytime. Patients in private rooms often have unrestricted visiting hours. But be aware of the fine line between offering assistance and taking up residence. Visitors should leave when the "visiting hours are over" announcement is made. When the hospital grows quieter, the patients get ready for sleep. If you intend to spend the night, speak with the nurse in charge.

  Notes: If your loved one cannot speak, never talk across him as though he cannot hear. To be ignored makes one a "non-person." Hearing is the last sense we lose.

  Keep conversations cheerful, speak softly and sit quietly when the person is asleep. Continue conversation with a friend in the visitors' waiting room. Leave children and animals at home.

  Comforting gestures such as a hug, kiss or pat makes one feel loved and appreciated. However, use discretion with more intimate contact. A hospital room is open to hospital staff, a roommate and visitors. Intimacy requires privacy and makes observers uncomfortable.

- **Meals and special diets**

  When the doctor has ordered nothing by mouth (NPO), and food is taken by mistake, tests may need to be canceled and rescheduled. Never bring food or drinks for your loved one unless approved by the doctor or nurse in charge. Save the candy for a "homecoming gift" unless the person is on a regular diet.

Do not eat food from a patient's plate. The amount of food eaten is recorded and adequate food is important for his recovery. If the patient does not eat, a liquid supplement may be offered. In most hospitals, a visitor may order a tray for themselves, may eat in the hospital cafeteria, where prices are reasonable and the food is well-prepared, or visit vending machines. Worried family members sometimes forget to eat and may drink far too much coffee.

- **Clothing and Linens**
  Those unflattering, open-backed hospital gowns are made of cotton and are surprisingly comfortable. They absorb perspiration and damp gowns are easily changed. If personal clothes are permitted, they should be laundered at home. Clothes made of 50/50 or 100% cotton are more comfortable to wear. The hospital does not assume responsibility for lost clothes. Storage space is limited.

Note: Do not bring heating pads, electric blankets or special pillows without permission from the nurse in charge. If an item is approved, the patient will be asked to sign a release form.

- **Valuables and Money**
  Leave jewelry at home, except for a watch and wedding band that fits well. If it is loose, there is a danger of losing the ring or if the finger swells, it may need to be removed. A patient may ask to wear their wedding ring during surgery. The doctor may approve and place tape over it.

  A small amount of money may be kept in the bedside table for small purchases such as the newspaper or stationery. A hospital admission kit contains several basic items but deodorant, toothpaste, etc., may be brought from home.

- **Supplemental Remedies**
  Do not bring medicines, laxatives or aspirin from home. The

doctor must know exactly what the patient has taken. The same rule applies for alcoholic beverages. Inform the nurse in charge if over-the-counter drugs or home remedies have been used routinely at home.

- **General Information, More Rules**
  - The patient living in a strange hospital room needs his or her glasses, hearing aids, dentures and cane. Without good vision and hearing, it is easy to become disoriented and fearful. The patient needs to wear his dentures if he is alert.

  - Many hospital rooms are furnished with lounge chairs for the patient's use when out of bed. When not in use, family members may enjoy them.

  - The "egg crate" (dimpled, foam mattress pad) is routinely ordered when the patient will spend most of the time in bed. It adds comfort, protects the skin and relieves pressure under bony joints. If not ordered by the doctor, the patient or a family member may request one when necessary. The pad and the contents of the admission kit may be taken home when the patient is discharged, because they are included in the hospital charges.

    At home, the pad may be placed in the bath tub as a cushion, cut into a square to pad a chair seat or placed on a slippery floor for the person to step on when getting out of a bed or chair. The pad can be washed on a gentle cycle and dried with cool air.

  - Do not sit on the hospital bed unless the patient asks you to sit closer. The patient may be uncomfortable if the bed is shaken, a traction might shift if one side of the mattress is depressed or the covers may be restricted by you.

— Patients look forward to having visitors as they recover. Cards, books, magazines, crafts or small games offer a change from endless television. Your days may seem hectic, but remember that time passes slowly for a recovering loved one.

— Other common rules:

   1. Visitors should use a visitor's bathroom and not the patient's bathroom which is usually shared with a roommate or next-door neighbors.

   2. Smoke only in designated areas and never around oxygen. Oxygen supports combustion and remains in the bed clothes for several hours after being turned off.

   3. Use both soap and water when you wash your hands. Cover your nose and mouth when you cough or sneeze. Do not expose patients to unwanted viruses.

— Let the nursing staff handle soiled bed linens. If you help change the bed, roll linens into a loose ball and hold them away from your clothes. Wash your hands afterwards.

— Do not enter a busy nurses' station, linen or supply room. Do not place food or other items in the refrigerator nor take any drinks out of it.

— Do not "tip" hospital personnel for the care given. If you are appreciative, send a note to the nursing service office after your loved one is discharged. Mention any staff members who have given excellent care. A box of candy for the hospital staff is a thoughtful gesture.

The doctors, nurses and social workers are aware that a loved one's stay is stressful for his family and friends. Family members may find it difficult to leave the seriously ill person. They may become exhausted and irritable, worry over the unexpected financial burden, or remain overly optimistic about the amount of recovery possible.

Comment: When I step inside the hospital doors, I do not see a maze of halls, rooms, people hurrying by or notice the pager's voice. I see a building with protective walls where miracles happen. I am aware that to many people the hospital is an alien place. One friend told me he feels like a "bull in a china shop," uncomfortable and out of place. Perhaps by understanding the rules, you will feel a little like I do.

Solving Problems During a Hospital Stay

Making Decisions

If the patient is conscious and capable of assuming responsibility for decision making, the members of the medical team will discuss with the patient his medical condition, the treatment choices available and the anticipated outcome of each choice. The doctor will recommend a course of treatment and answer questions. The patient is now prepared to make an "informed" decision.

When the patient is unconscious, a responsible person must act in his behalf. The guardian should make all decisions as the helpless person would want them made. The guardian has an obligation to learn the facts and consider the consequences of decisions made.

Misunderstandings and Other Incidents

Who does the family speak to if they believe the patient has been neglected or mistreated? Turn to the nurses.

Be sure you understand what has actually happened. You should learn the names of those involved, the time of day, and the specifics concerning the incident. Even if you suspect that the patient has misunderstood, speak with the nurse in charge. Ask that she explain and clear up any misunderstanding with the patient. Peace of mind and trust in hospital caregivers are important to the patient's recovery.

If you grow concerned and suspect that more than a misunderstanding is involved, start by speaking with the nurse in charge. Listen to the explanations and solutions offered.

If the patient believes that more should be done to correct the problem, speak next with nursing administration (Assistant Director, Patient Relations Coordinator or Advocate). Explain what has happened and to whom you have spoken.

You or your loved one may discuss the incident with the doctor at any time. However, if it is a nursing care problem, you may wish to give nursing service an opportunity to correct it. At any rate, the doctor should be informed.

Before Discharge from the Hospital

Patients are being discharged earlier today and will spend more time recuperating at home. Before the day of discharge, you should ask the doctor:

- Will special equipment, specific exercises or a special diet be needed at home?

- What conditions or possible complications should I watch for?

- What kind of recovery can we expect?

Physical therapists, inhalation therapists and registered dietitians are members of the hospital staff, and each specialist will provide information if asked. You may need to know how equipment works, how to regulate and how to clean it. Exercises may be ordered or a special diet prescribed. Use this opportunity to gain valuable information.

The social worker or discharge planner is a problem solver who will help put you and your loved one in touch with community resources and support groups. Some of the problems you may wish to discuss are:

- Limited financial resources

- Your loved one's emotional problems

- Transportation to treatment centers

- Needed assistance with housekeeping or nursing care

- Guidelines for government programs - such as Medicare, Medicaid, SSI, etc.

You will find social workers interested, involved and knowledgeable. They understand how to work within the framework of the medical system, and keep the person from "falling through the cracks." In general, the medical staff will be very supportive. You must add the fragments of information you receive to your present knowledge. Continue to ask questions until you understand how best to help your loved one.

Chapter Thirteen

WHEN YOU CAN NO LONGER PROVIDE CARE ALONE

The needs of a disabled loved one dictate the type of care he should receive. If the condition changes, so do his needs. The caregiver may need assistance and later her patient may require skilled or professional care. This chapter describes the type of help available in most communities and discusses the steps in decision making.

One of man's greatest strengths is the ability to adapt. The members of a family will adapt to the changing needs of their disabled loved one. Their lives continue in an orderly routine until one day the caregiver realizes that a change is needed.

My son managed to care for his daily needs while I worked 10 minutes away. He rode the bus for disabled and seniors to his appointments for physical therapy. Although improvement was minimal, the ongoing chemotherapy treatments seemed to control the erratic cancer growth. We hoped for another remission.

While driving to work one morning, I considered how well my son was meeting his daily needs, given his failing strength. By the time I parked the car, I had decided to search for someone who would provide care while I was gone. I could not identify how his condition had changed, but sensed that he needed some assistance. And he did.

How does one know that it is time to reevaluate the situation?

- You are aware that the person's needs have changed or gradually increased, and you consider if he requires more support or skilled care than you are capable of giving.

- You are exhausted and need help. The respite caregiver can no longer help you, for instance.
  The promised assistance from family and friends has been undependable.

- The doctor concludes that your loved one needs a new treatment or other care which requires skilled nursing.

These and other problems, such as increasing anger and conflict, should trigger a discussion with the disabled person. You may both agree that it is time to learn more about the alternative care available in your community. Start your search by speaking with a social worker in Social Services, a discharge planner at the hospital or a counselor at the Division on Aging.

Note: When someone requires additional or more skilled care, the increased cost may soon deplete his resources. At this time he may qualify for assistance from government programs. All qualified counselors are familiar with resource guidelines. As discussed, it is the disabled person's financial resources that are evaluated, not yours, and when his finances are depleted, the patient may qualify for various government programs.

Community resources include:

- **Home Care Services**
  A full-service home health care agency should coordinate and provide any level of care, from treatment by professional nurses or therapists to personal and respite care. The agency should be certified by Medicare, Medicaid and possibly the

Joint Commission for Accreditation of Home Care Organizations. Check with the local office of the Division on Aging. Don't be concerned whether the agency is non-profit, hospital-related, part of a national chain, or small and independent. You are concerned with the staff's ability to provide good care. The cost per hour is determined by the level of the caregivers skills. Average rates for various levels of caregivers:

Nurse practitioners and register nurses . . . . . $50-$100/Hr.
Practical or vocational nurses, Licensed rehabilitative
  therapists, Geriatric social workers. . . . . $35-$ 75/Hr.
Home health aides . . . . $10-$ 20/Hr.
Homemakers, companions. . . . . $ 7-$ 15/Hr.

Always ask about other (hidden) charges. For instance, is there a minimum charge per visit or a higher cost for night or weekend care? Evaluations are usually included in the fee, but inquire. Ask for the names of several clients that you may contact as references.

Community agencies may have home care services also, which may be offered on a sliding scale rate, the lower the income, the lower the rate. The one needing the services may be married, in which case the joint husband/wife income minus certain standardized deductions, will determine the total income. Ask the counselor to review the financial picture.

- **Other Supplemental Services**
  — Meals on Wheels
    Brings hot, tasty, ready-to-eat food to the home five days each week for an easily affordable fee. Extra food is provided for weekend meals.

  — Transportation and Escort Service
    Community groups and agencies often provide free

transportation, usually with wheelchair access, to senior centers, shopping malls, libraries and for medical appointments. If asked, the service may provide escorts to accompany the disabled people for assistance and greater safety on the street.

— Housekeeping and Grocery Services
State and local agencies or volunteer groups will offer low cost (or free) part-time housekeepers or grocery shoppers for the low income disabled or elderly.

— Companion Service
Volunteers will schedule regular visits each week. They do not provide care, but offer conversation, humor and companionship without a fee. Church groups may offer this service.

— Telephone Safety Service
A phone call at the same time each day provides reassurance for those living alone. LIFELINE, available in many places, provides an emergency response service which connects the disabled to a hospital or other emergency service. The line is connected to the phone for a nominal cost.

- **Adult Day Care and Respite Care**

— Adult Day-Care Centers
The disabled or elderly person may spend a full day or a half day in a center which offers medical care, meals, companionship, naps and other activities. The center, if affiliated with a hospital, may offer screening and rehabilitative services. Regular attendance may be a requirement.

The fees will vary according to the services offered and how the center has been funded. Adult day-care centers will permit the caregiver to continue working and will provide activities and protection for the disabled person who attends. Fees are usually very reasonable.

— Respite Care
Respite care workers offer the caregiver some free time. They may be available for a few hours on a regular basis, for a weekend or for a week or more. Employees and volunteers of various community organizations can provide the level of expertise needed. The cost is reasonable and in some cases, may be free unless the care is provided by a medical facility.

Note: Other community programs which may prove valuable for you and your loved one include:

Senior Centers
Offer hot meals, organized activities, informal companionship and some respite care on a drop-in basis, at no cost.

City and county health clinics
Public Health offers regular health monitoring and screenings which are free or low cost.

Community agencies
Offer home care education programs. Check with the American Red Cross and local hospitals.

Support groups
Meet weekly or monthly and offer the disabled, their caregiver and family an opportunity to discuss various problems, share solutions and investigate new treatments, while enjoying the association with others who have faced similar problems.

Finding Help in Decision Making

Networking, an overused word, is very appropriate for your efforts. Find people who are well informed about the programs in your area. Ask for suggestions of whom to contact and the names of key personnel. You may be surprised to learn how many programs offer help to meet your loved one's needs. Many are staffed by dedicated, trained volunteers who strive to help their neighbors.

It takes determination and effort to locate all the assistance available in your community. You should question if your loved one is eligible for these programs based on his present income and if not, what the cost will be. Your efforts may allow your loved one to remain at home and as the caregiver, you will have assistance and freedom.

If you cannot evaluate your loved one's needs, do not have time to search for resources and are willing to pay for the service, contact a private Care Manager. A manager is a professional counselor (nurse, social worker) who will assess the person's long term needs and organize support services. You will find the manager knowledgeable about the quality of the care available and willing to locate difficult to find services. To locate a list of Care Managers, check the yellow pages under the heading, "Older Adult Care Managers" or "Geriatric Management." You may also ask the doctor.

Questions to ask before hiring a Care Manager:

- What is your professional background and where have you worked locally?
  He or she should have a license or degree in Public Health Nursing, social work or extensive experience in nursing, geriatrics or health management.

- What are your fees and what does that include?
  Some managers charge an initial fee for a home visit and evaluation, plus an hourly charge of $15-$100 while making arrangements and for follow-up visits. Some funded

programs offer free or low-cost counseling to low-income families.

- What continuing support do you offer?
  Ask if the manager is available for phone calls, emergencies or visits.

  - How are problem situations handled?

  - May we contact one or more of your clients for a reference?

Sign the agreement when the services and fees are spelled out. Remain informed and involved in future decision making.

An Example of Assistance Planning:

- Three mornings a week — from 8 until 12 noon an aide will assist with personal care, etc.

- One afternoon a week — a companion visits to give you free time.

- Noon one day a week — have lunch at the Senior Center. Stay to play cards or other games. You will accompany him and attend a program.

- One hour every three weeks — a nurse changes the catheter and checks the person's condition.

- Once a week — a housekeeper helps with cleaning.

- Respite care — a long weekend is planned every two months.

- Two friends have agreed to visit on alternate Wednesday evenings so that you may attend your favorite club meeting or church.

- Sunday mornings, two church members will stop by to take your loved one, with his wheelchair, to church.

- One son, who lives nearby, has invited the family to dinner every two weeks. Though busy, he reminds you that he is always available to help you.

- A daughter who lives some distance away, has agreed to write regularly, to transfer favorite old records onto cassettes and has made plans to visit in the near future.

These arrangements will give you 20-24 hours per week of free time when others provide care. The total help employed per week:

> Aide = three visits = 12 hours a week
> RN = one visit for one hour every three weeks
> Housekeeper = 3-4 hours a week if available

The Move Outside the Home

Arrangements must be made when the present care does not meet a loved one's needs or when you have become exhausted or ill. The loved one should be involved in the decision making, if mentally alert, for it involves his future.

When one can no longer remain at home, even with support services, you as the caregiver, should call a conference with the loved ones. You may phone or write and, with luck, they may meet around the dining table. Each one should clearly understand the loved one's present condition and how the situation has changed. This is a time for gentle persuasion, consideration for others' feelings and loving concern for a loved one's future.

A painful decision is made more difficult when those involved cannot agree. In most instances, a mother, daughter or daughter-in-law has been the primary caregiver, with other family members providing respite support. When a change must be made, however, everyone may want equal decision-making rights. Sometimes the person offering the least support, personal or financial, may become the most adamant that the loved one remain at home.

Comments such as "I promised her that she could stay in her home until she died," "How can you give up and let her be taken care of by strangers?" express strong feelings. A child may deny that the person's condition has deteriorated. If others feel they have been neglectful, their guilt may influence their words.

How to Present the Situation

- Gently explain to your loved one the reality of the present situation. If the person is capable of understanding and sharing in the decision making, describe the options. The doctor may be the one who explains the alternatives for home care. Allow time for the person to understand and accept the need for change.

- When you contact the other family members or those involved in a final decision, explain the situation clearly and reasonably. State what the doctor has recommended and ask for their suggestions. Try to act as the catalyst who keeps communications open.

- Consider each choice that is available. Before viewing the nursing home as a "last resort" choice, visit those nearby and evaluate them objectively.

- Try to make the final decision together. If your loved one's health improves, other options will be considered. If family members cannot agree and remain inflexible and unhappy, your loved one still deserves the quality care that you can no longer provide. Consult the doctor and together, the three of you should make the final decision.

Checksheet For Nursing Homes, Other Facilities

When you visit a center, check items by rating 1 (excellent) 2 (good) 3 (fair) 4 (poor), or answer questions with Yes or No. Be observant and expect answers to all questions.

	#1	#2	#3
Name of Center			
Located near your home			
Located on a bus route			
Clean, comfortable, cheerful			
Free of offensive odors			
Rooms are light and cheery			
Adequate storage, sink in room			
Shared or private bath			
General attitude of staff			
Prompt attention to needs			
Food appearance and variety, quantity served, temperature			

Questions to Ask:

1. Does the admission contract state costs, services provided, discharge conditions, refunds?

2. Can the guardian with power of attorney see the chart anytime?

3. Are relatives notified immediately in case of injury?

4. Does the resident have a choice of pharmacies?

5. Can the family bring over-the-counter items (aspirin, etc.?)

6. Are mealtime visits O.K.?

7. Are restraints used (physical or chemical) without a doctor's order?

8. Is a care plan followed and can the family see it?

9. May the family
     visit anytime?   ___________   ___________   ___________

Other questions:
  How are roommates
     selected?   ___________   ___________   ___________

  What is the daily schedule and what
     are the planned activities? ___________   ___________   ___________

  What personal possessions may be brought?
  A favorite chair, TV or radio?___________   ___________   ___________

Comments:

(1) ____

   ____

   ____

(2) ____

   ____

   ____

(3) ____

   ____

   ____

Condensed from a Facility Comparison Checklist prepared by Senior Advocates, Inc., Worchester, Mass.
(The checksheet may be enlarged when Xeroxed.)

Suggestions for Selecting an Extended Care Facility

You should review several books on nursing homecare in the library.

As a former Nursing Director, I wish to add a more personal viewpoint to help you in decision making.

The nursing home administration must comply with federal regulations. Nursing assistants employed by the center must have completed a standardized course of training and be certified. A resident may choose his doctor and his pharmacy. A state-employed ombudsman is a patient's advocate who will investigate patient's complaints and help mediate problems.

Note: Check with the State Department of Human Services and their nursing home division for more answers. You may wish to ask about the punitive record of the homes before you select one.

The quality of caregiving by the staff has to do with the less tangible aspects of care, such as the center's policies, the knowledge, concern and organizational ability of the supervising personnel plus the attitudes and abilities of the actual caregivers. The hiring practices and the demand for accountability by the nursing administration directly influence the type of care a loved one receives. Any problems should be taken to the supervising nurse or nurse administrator.

How do you determine the type of care being given? Once you have asked the questions on your check list, use your eyes, ears and good common sense. Try to time one visit on a Friday evening during the meal. If you are acquainted with a resident pay a visit. If not, walk through the center as if you were visiting.

Listen to the tone of voice and the responses by the staff. Even when a patient is hard of hearing and the caregiver speaks loudly, she should smile and speak kindly. Listen for impatient comments or snide remarks for they let you know how the speaker feels. Note if a patient is ignored. Watch the residents' faces and consider how comfortable they appear to be with members of the staff.

You will gain an overall impression of the center, which has less to do with a lovely living room and more to do with a kind, helpful atmosphere. Keep in mind that this is the residents' home, usually their only home, where they spend most of the time.

A capable staff will treat even the most confused patient with respect, will answer repeated questions, will tolerate beliefs and idiosyncrasies and will share the humor of funny situations. They should feel responsible for the resident's well-being. Because of this involvement, the patient's feeling of loneliness and isolation diminishes. The minor complaints to loved ones may continue, however, for some residents wish to remind others that this is not their home, and the move was not of their choosing.

Many centers encourage children's and animal's visits and permit the residents' rooms to be decorated with plants and personal treasures. Rows of rocking chairs may be lined up on a covered patio or front porch. The picture I have painted may be an ideal one, but use it for comparison as you inspect centers.

It is my belief that a well-run nursing home with a capable staff offers several advantages that elderly residents may not find elsewhere:

A world of their own. The pace is slow, food is familiar and the emphasis is on flexibility and accommodation in meeting residents' medical and physical needs. Special considerations, such as pots of fresh-brewed coffee are waiting at six each morning for early risers, corn bread and other favorite foods are added to the menu at residents' request and concerns about aches, pains and elimination are taken seriously, all help make a center a home. Little kindnesses create a warm, friendly place. The residents are protected from the hectic, changing pace of the everyday world and its harsher aspects where helplessness may make someone a potential victim.

A place where shared memories have importance. It seems more difficult to form close friendships as we grow older, but the companionship of lively discussions about the years gone by, such as a first airplane ride, a 200 mile trip that was an event and took all day and entertainment that revolved around a church social or family gathering, brings back fond memories. The residents have lived in a gentler, slower-paced world unknown to young people today and to a degree, they have found it again. Pleasant hours are spent visiting, playing checkers or dominoes, working on hobbies or napping for awhile. The younger residents may find the seniors to be polite, interested and supportive.

When you have selected one or two centers, try to visit one more time. If you choose an evening, remember that evening meals should be light. With a smaller staff in the evening, observe how quickly the patients' lights and requests are being answered. Most of the staff members should remain to care for patients' needs as one or two of the staff take a break.

Note: Any center, or home for that matter, may have a localized, unpleasant odor which will be dissipated by a deodorizing spray. It is the generalized foul and sour odor that lingers throughout the building that should cause a visitor to question how quickly residents incontinence has been cleaned up. The handling and storage of soiled linens may add to the foul odor. Well-run centers do not have this problem.

As I write, many charming stories come to mind, but I will recount only one or maybe two.

The staff believed that a new resident was a busybody for she seemed to move in and out of others' rooms during the day. One day I decided to check on her activities. During the morning, she wrote a letter for one lady who had severe arthritis, brushed and braided another's hair and read a chapter of a book to a third. After lunch she pushed a man in a wheelchair near the patio window because he asked to sit in the sun. Later, I saw her sitting with her neighbor as they both napped in adjourning chairs with handiwork in their laps. So much for our suspected gossip.

A short elderly gentleman wore garters on the sleeve of his white shirt and a brown felt hat. He was very hard of hearing and as a consequence, he spoke in a loud voice. He would walk down the hall and ask the nurse, "Now, where am I going?"

During the day, the staff reminded him that he was going to lunch, for coffee, to sit on the patio, etc. I met him one time and suggested that he "was going" to watch TV. I helped him to be seated and as I turned to leave the room, I heard this booming voice behind me say, "Now where am I going?" I could understand how upsetting this would be to his family as I laughed and ask a nursing assistant to help him. Incidentally, this was the man who would not come to breakfast one morning because he could not find his teeth. His nurse located the missing dentures under the bed lying inside his felt hat. The arrangement had seemed logical to him.

Chapter Fourteen

WHEN A LOVED ONE'S LIFE IS ENDING

Death is a part of our life's cycle. The caregiver and other loved ones, though sad, have an opportunity to help the person work out the loose ends of his life and to find a sense of closure. With hospice care, the staff and volunteers support the loved one as well as his family. This chapter discusses hospice care, spending the final days at home, signs of approaching death and finally, grief and the recovery process.

Hospice Care

The word Hospice means, "A shelter or way station for travelers on their journey," and was chosen to symbolically describe a place where one might rest as he nears the end of his life. A hospice is best described in the words of hospice nurses and volunteers:

"When doctors decide that nothing more can be done, the patient's life can often be measured in months, not years. The person is hurting, lonely and scared. We stop their pain and help them and their family improve the quality of the rest of their life."

"He now has the freedom to do whatever he wants. Realizing that he may be doing something for the last time brings a special enjoyment."

"Families are in pain when a loved one is in pain. Freedom from pain returns the loved one's dignity and relieves the family's agony."

"As hospice volunteers, we share a special time in their life, often becoming the bridge over which they and their family can share a new closeness and acceptance of death."

"We are the non-judgmental listener who permits honest, meaningful conversations. When our patient and his loved ones are able to find a sense of closure in their relationships, they have a sense of peace. The person finds more meaning in the life he has lived."

"Hospice care continues after a loved one's death with unconditional love and support for those suffering the loss."

My sister, Wanda Stokes, an RN and experienced hospice volunteer, has an expertise in pain control, grief counseling and the process of dying. Terminally ill patients and their families are recipients of the unique care and support provided by hospice staffs and volunteers. Hospice care is available for any terminally ill person who asks. It is sad that many seek support only days before their death, and sadder still if their doctor fails to suggest hospice care when the person chooses to spend his final weeks or months at home.

The comparison between traditional hospital care and hospice care is that the emphasis has shifted.

Traditional Care

- Death is denied and a cure is searched for at all costs.

- The emphasis is placed on the disease process and the new technology available.

- A sense of defeat is felt when nothing more can be done, and the treatment is considered a medical failure.

- The terminal patient may be isolated from those expected to live, and may have fewer opportunities to share time with family and friends.

Note: Traditional care is exactly what one wants and expects when he enters the hospital. It is only during the final, terminal stage of his life that the emphasis changes.

Hospice Care

- Death is viewed as a part of the life cycle. The goal is now not to shorten life, but rather avoid prolonging it.

- Emphasis is on the patient as a person, not a disease, and is geared toward supportive care and freedom from discomfort.

- Emphasis is on the quality of life during the time remaining.

- Communication and support are stressed. Families assume the caregiving role (with support from volunteers). Hospice workers help the terminal person and the loved ones resolve any unfinished business in their lives.

You may have expected the diagnosis, but feel sad and at times, angry, before the shock ends and the acceptance of your future loss begins. It is a time for questions before decisions.

Has the person been told? If not, why not?
Is he or she capable of assisting with decision making?
Will I be able to care for him if he wants to come home?
If not, where will I find help?

If your loved one is enrolled in hospice, a registered nurse will evaluate his condition, the amount of pain and the general care needed; then will design a plan for care. Hospice volunteers may assist with personal care, household tasks, or respite care (so you may have a few hours relief and free time). Professional nurses will determine the effectiveness of pain control, will observe for complications and will evaluate the person's changing needs. You need not be alone as death approaches unless you choose to be.

Guidelines for Hospice Care

- Hospice may be aligned with a community hospital, be a free-standing hospice center or remain an independent community program.

- A patient will sign into the program for 90 days and be re-evaluated (for continuing care) at the end of that time.

- The patient has his or her own physician. Nurses coordinate the care, evaluate needs during home visits and maintain the same level of doctor-nurse communication and record keeping as with hospitalized patients. The patient will not be admitted to the hospital except for complications which require hospital treatment. Patients may be admitted for a short stay to evaluate and adjust medications or to give their caregivers a respite.

- If at any time, the patient and his family decide to pursue aggressive medical treatment instead of hospice care, the agreement with hospice ends and the patient leaves hospice care. He may be readmitted, but must wait until the end of the 90-day enrollment period.

- Included with hospice care is the equipment needed in the home, medications (ordered by the doctor) and necessary supplies.

- Most hospice care is Medicare and Medicaid approved and their standards for payment are followed (with a ceiling on physician's services). Other sources of payment for services are private insurance, the patient or the hospice. The non-profit hospice programs welcome financial gifts so that no one will be denied hospice care that requests and needs it.

These comments from the hospice training program define it:

We have stopped treating the disease; it has won. Now we treat the symptoms so the patient can be pain-free, alert, and able to enjoy each day left.

Our goal is to help transfer control and power back to the patient.

Controlling pain is the first priority. If pain is under control, there are no thoughts of suicide. The fear of recurring pain influences the pain experienced, so medication should be given routinely. The frequency may change, but medication should not stop even if the person becomes semi-conscious.

When we face death, we consider our faith and belief in eternity. Caregivers should keep their beliefs out of the conversation, so the person can find his own God.

Always listen. The more one can express his feelings, the better he can evaluate himself.

Give considerate, honest answers to questions. If the person is afraid that information will be hidden from him, remind him that, "What we know, you'll know."

When the patient feels that his life is worth living, death holds less fear.

If loved ones have had an opportunity to grieve in anticipation of death and remain nearby as death approaches, they will realize that death arrives gently. They will also experience a sense of closure.

Care of the Terminally Ill Loved One at Home

The terminally ill loved one usually wants to return to the security of familiar surroundings. As you make plans to help him end his life peacefully, in comfort and with dignity at home, consider these suggestions:

- Keep the room well lighted and well ventilated and use a night light so he will not awaken in a dark room. As the body becomes weaker, vision may be poorer.

- He may feel more comfortable lying on his back, with the head slightly elevated and with a soft pillow under the knees. Help him turn on his side every few hours for a short while. Support the back while on his side with a pillow placed lengthwise against it. Place a small pillow between the knees.

- Use lightweight covers to keep uncomfortable pressure off the toes. The room may feel cooler to someone lying in bed than to you, who are active. Small comforters add warmth.

- Speak in a normal voice and do not talk across a loved one if he seems to be semi-conscious. Hearing is the last sense lost.

- Give a warm sponge bath daily. Use soap sparingly, rinse well and pat dry. Give a gentle and not vigorous backrub to relax tired muscles. Sprinkle baby powder over back, buttocks, under breast and in skin folds. Tighten the bottom sheet to remove any uncomfortable wrinkles.

- If the person has little appetite, encourage him to sip liquid supplements (Ensure) and drink water. When nourishment or water can no longer be taken, wash the face and hands with a warm, moist washcloth and give ice chips with a spoon or let him suck on hard candy.

- Check the back, hips and heels for any skin breakdown. Place a pad ("egg crate" foam, polyester sheepskin, or air mattress) on top of the mattress. Add a disposable pad under the hips.

- If he is unable to speak, ask questions that can be answered with a nod or shake of the head and explain what you plan to do. Be sure that any pain is well controlled.

- Be aware of elimination. The urine output will diminish with less fluid intake, but a full, distended bladder makes one restless and uncomfortable. Severe constipation or an impaction can cause a headache, nausea and vomiting.

  Note: A recent study has determined that a terminally ill person shouldn't be given food and water artificially if he doesn't want it, because it may only heighten discomfort. Starving seems to ease one's death,

> since dehydration lessons consciousness, promotes sleepiness and diminishes pain, the researchers reported. Most want very little nourishment during their final months. Those with cancer generally do not experience hunger, and if they do, a small amount of food satisfies them. If thirsty, they suck ice chips or hard candy.

Dr. Robert McMann states that family members and doctors may insist they must give nourishment artificially when they don't know what to do for we equate food with love. When the terminal person was allowed to have anything he wanted, he consumed less than 25% of the food or liquids needed for normal nutritional requirements.

Near Death Awareness

Hospice nurses are aware that people who are slowly dying may develop a "nearing death awareness," a special knowledge of what dying and death are like. They may realize what they need in order to die peacefully. If their loved ones will listen carefully, they may understand the dying person's comments and requests.

Often the attempt to describe what is happening during the process of dying or to express a final request is missed, misunderstood or ignored. The comments may be obscure, expressed in symbolic talk or related to a personal experience. Don't automatically assume that they are confused or "losing their mind."

Facing Death Together

When the symptoms of approaching death are visible, ask other family members or close friends to be near and lend support. The symptoms are the result of a circulatory and metabolic slowdown and may include one or more of the following:

- The arms and legs feel cold to the touch.

- The skin appears white with a grayish tinge.

- The respirations become more irregular and shallow, with a complete stop for 10-30 seconds at a time.

- The mouth may relax and be open, and a rattle in the throat is heard. The ears will flatten against the head.

- The person may lapse into unconsciousness.

- You will become aware of a gentle "slipping away" from life.

No one wishes to die alone. We would prefer that someone hold our hand and quietly tell us to go toward the "light." The moment of death is a gentle, pain-free experience. Those who share this quiet moment may be saddened to lose a loved one but will experience a sense of closure, and may feel relieved that all suffering has ended.

Comment: A loved one may be upset that he or she had left the room just before the person died. It seems that when a mourning loved one is overly distraught and is having difficulty accepting the approaching death, the person whose life is ending may wait until the grieving loved one has left the room before dying.

Understanding the Dying

An experienced nurse states that to die prematurely is an oxymoron when dealing with terminal patients. She explained:

"We all choose how, when, and where we leave our bodies. Therefore all deaths take place at the right time... Our patients possess the power to die - or the will to live. We are just witnesses."

(From "Insights on Death and Dying," Nursing 95 Journal, January)

As Death Approaches

The changes due to approaching death may be recognizable. The body does not function as it has before. You may notice only one or two of the indicators of approaching death, but usually they are seen in combination.

Changes

Circulation slows. Arms and legs may feel cool to the touch.

Metabolism changes. May sleep for longer periods, more difficult to waken. May grow restless and pick at bed linens. Needs less food and drinks.

Secretions may thicken in the back of the throat (you may hear a rattle).

Breathing may become irregular, with 10-30 second periods of no breathing.

May have a loss of control. Bladder may lose urine and anal sphincter may relax as death approaches.

Vision may become dim and blurred. Hearing is the last sense to diminish.

What To Do

Keep warm with blankets (not electric blanket)

Stay with loved one when he is most alert, speak in calm, confident tones (do not startle). Mention who you are. Wash the face and hands with a warm, moist washcloth. Pat dry.

Start a cool mist-humidifier in the room. Give ice chips, sips of water through a straw.

Elevate the head to help them breath more easily.

Pad the bed with extra disposable pads to prevent the linen changes.

Leave lights on, continue to speak and reassure them of your presence. Never assume they cannot hear you.

Messages of the Dying

Naomi Feil in her book, *Validation,* discusses how the "old, old" person is still working out past problems and painful experiences. He or she may appear confused and incoherent, but they are viewing old memories in their mind's eye. They are validating their life.

The messages of the dying seem intertwined with the loved ones who are being left behind and others who have died previously. The words may not make sense to their loved ones, until they listen more carefully. Two experienced nurses, Patricia Kelly and Maggie Callahan, state that they find patients approaching death either at ease or "busy" in a purposeful way. We have them to thank for sharing the following experiences:

An 81-year-old-lady was cared for by her husband, Joe. Her only daughter, Susan, had died the previous year and she was concerned about leaving her husband alone. She had become withdrawn, distant and seldom wanted to talk. The nurse asked, "Laura, what's happening to you? Where are you, dear?" and she answered, "It's time to get in line."

The nurse never questioned the line's existence. "Tell me about the line. Is there anyone there you know?"

Smiling, she replied, "Susan."

"How nice for you," the nurse answered, then asked, "Would you like to get in line? Is it OK? Tell me more."

The smile faded. "But Joe can't go with me." It was the heart of her dilemma.

"That must be a hard choice for you. Can we help get Joe ready for the time you have to get in line?" "Yes," she sighed.

The nurse repeated the exact conversation to Joe, who wept, but took comfort in the realization that Laura was looking forward to being with Susan. He explained that the couple had traveled frequently, and had stood in many lines. She was getting ready for a solo voyage, was caught up in the struggle of whether to stay or go, and needed "permission" to die.

Joe understood, explained some plans he was considering, reassured her he would be all right and gave her the "permission" she needed. She became peaceful and remained so until she died two weeks later.

Another young man began asking, "Where am I? How do I get home? If I could find a map, I could get home."

His parents believed his confusion was due to a move into a new room, and placed familiar things around him. He grew more agitated, until the parents realized that he was trying to find his new home. Fighting their grief, they reassured him that he would find his way soon and that they were now ready for him to leave. His anxiety drained away and he died the next day.

Many people who are dying seem to have a glimpse of another world. They refer to a dream, or feel they are in another place. One man said, "I can see the light down the road, and it's beautiful." It was the one coherent moment that he had during his last 24 hours.

A person may talk to someone who has died, then listen for their response. It is like hearing a one-sided telephone conversation.

They may also talk to a mother or father who have died.

At times, the person approaching death seems to choose when to die. They seem to wait to see a loved one again, to have a first glimpse of a newborn or until a marriage or other happy event is over. They may seem to wait until someone leaves the room, wait until others arrive to support a grieving loved one or pick an appropriate moment so others may continue with planned events.

One lady told the hospice nurse that she would be gone so as to not interfere with a son's long-awaited trip and was buried one week before he was scheduled to leave. Another lady survived long enough to share the happiness of seeing her first great-grandchild.

During my son's last hospital stay, I phoned his stepfather who was on a disaster assignment in Guam. Although I had not considered this hospital admission more serious than others, something in my conversation alerted my husband. He sent word the next day that he was on the first flight to California. The following morning I was told that my son might not live through the day. That evening, after we had changed his bed, he was resting quietly when the bedside phone rang. My husband had arrived at the airport and as we were talking, I turned and watched my son take his final breath. My sister, Wanda, commented, "Perhaps he waited until you were not alone."

Maggie and Patricia mention another patient who gave the message that she was about to die. The young girl called her father to tell him that she loved him, and to thank him for being such a good father. He told her he was coming to see her after work. She replied, "I need to tell you now. I won't be able to then." Since her condition seemed stable and friends would be visiting, he assumed she meant they would not be alone. His daughter was in a coma when he arrived, and died that night. But in her own way, she had said her good-bye.

The two nurses stress the importance of listening attentively to the dying. They explain how to communicate:

- Respond in ways that tell them you accept whatever they say or "see."

- Follow what they say by gently asking questions. Ask them to repeat their answers if you don't understand. You may say, "I'm not sure I follow you. Can you explain that a little more?"

- Support them, but don't keep pushing. If they are having difficulty "letting go," don't deny the problem. Let them know that you understand and offer to help.

- If other loved ones enter the room, repeat their comments accurately.

Hospice workers try to help the dying person with a peaceful, gentle death. When they stare into space and reach toward what they are "seeing," they are encouraged to "go" toward what they are seeing.

If you and other family members have accepted your loved one's imminent death, and are able to give permission, hold them and share the moments of death. You will experience a sense of acceptance and closure in your own life.

Coping With Grief

When loved ones die, it is their presence we miss. The voice and laughter are gone, leaving the house empty and quiet. Those left behind know this, but search for the essence of that person in the memories of friends and relatives. They may engage in one-sided conversations when they are alone.

Everyone grieves in his or her own way. The loss of someone who was valuable and cherished in our life brings intense emotional pain. The pain can seem frightening and overwhelming and may remain a constant companion.

Common Reactions to Loss

The first reactions of shock and denial are the body's built-in anesthesia to cushion the emotional blow. They fade with the realization that the loved one is gone. The finality of the loss brings sadness and tears.

Anger, a common expression of grief, may be directed at the people or circumstances the person holds responsible for his loss. Working through the anger often provides the energy needed to cope. A second response to grief is to blame one's self for something done or left undone before the loved one's death. Blame and guilt cloud the happy memories of special times together. The person should talk with a trusted friend. They need to be reminded that they are human and to forgive themselves.

In time, the strong emotions are spent, life seems to go on, but loneliness and depression may increase. The person feels that they mourn alone, withdrawing from their past social life. They find comfort in talking to the person who has died, and may believe they have heard the familiar voice. The grieving person may develop physical illnesses, be unable to sleep or eat, have headaches or feel exhausted.

It is about this time that the grieving loved one may have a panicky feeling, decide to move, quit a job, sell a house and change their life. It seems to them that the time has come to run away from painful memories and reminders. Those who love them should talk them out of it. Emptiness and loneliness will accompany them to a strange, new place. The greatest mourning often occurs about six months after the loss of a loved one. If the person will work through the grief in familiar surroundings (for perhaps a year), they will have time to make a less emotional and more business-like decision.

A grieving person is easily hurt and may be overly sensitive to real or imagined "slights." They may become angry with even the most sympathetic friends. Resentment and withdrawal will only increase the pain of loss. It is forgiveness, as the bitterness fades, that helps one heal.

Finally, the surviving loved one is afraid that their memories will fade and that others will forget. They begin to share their memories, and with the exchange, the store of happy memories grows. The feeling of depression may alternate with moments of optimism. Eventually, the person takes steps to become involved again. The loss has been accepted and memories become less painful as they go on with their life.

When we lose someone whom we have loved unconditionally, the pain is intense. We cannot move ahead with our future life until our grief work (with all its pain) is done. When grief is delayed or one does not move ahead after a time of mourning, the mourner may take on grief as a life style. The person may even suffer intense reactions months or years later when circumstances trigger flashbacks. Grief may be masked with a dependence on drugs, a growing anger toward friends and family or a rejection of offers of help.

There is not a normal length of time for grieving. Active grieving may continue up to three years or more. Most people usually begin to carry on regular activities after about six months to a year. Renewed feelings of grief and loss may be triggered by holidays or the anniversary of the death. It might be comforting to be with old friends during these times.

How to Help Yourself Through Grief

- Be kind to yourself. Some days and weeks will be more difficult than others. Remember that you will eventually recover.

- Talk about your feelings. Visit with those who make you feel comfortable and explain in your own way. Don't hold all the pain inside.

- Rest and exercise each day. Take small naps during the day and exercise to help control depression.

- Remember to eat. Eat small amounts of a variety of foods as often as you can tolerate food. Drink plenty of water and other drinks but avoid alcohol (a "downer") and limit caffeine.

- Consider your spiritual needs. When we lose a loved one we may question our beliefs, be angry with God and consider the meaning of life and death. Spiritual support helps us cope.

- Be aware of physical problems. If they seem to go beyond the normal effects of grieving, see your doctor.

- Ask for and accept help. During the moments when you are at a loss to make a decision or continue other responsibilities, let those you trust and who care about you help. Take "Call me if you need me" statements seriously. Friends will feel needed and helpful. They may help with shopping, household duties, phones, food or transportation. Finally, ask for professional help if your feelings of despair become overwhelming or if you have any thoughts of suicide.

Note: Loved ones who must cope with a sudden death such as suicide, sudden infant death or an accidental death, need support. The person grieving has special problems. The participants in a support group offer understanding and support based on their own experiences. Call the local hospice, mental health association or hospital for the name and phone number of support groups.

Children grieve over their loss in many of the same ways as adults, but are often unable to express their grief. Sometimes they are so overwhelmed by their grief, (or by the grief of others around them) that they repress their feelings. Adults may give the child confused messages: "Dad has gone on a long journey or mom has gone to sleep for a long while." In an attempt to protect them, the adult has isolated the child from the grieving process. They have discouraged them from talking about their loss. The child may fear that other loved ones will leave them. Adults who are observant may see children act out their grief in play or in anti-social behavior.

Take time to calm and reassure the child with affection and physical comfort. Explain briefly, truthfully, and in a simple way what has happened. They may ask for more information later. Let children express their feelings. Reassure them that anything they did, said, or wished done did not cause the death. Children may be encouraged (but never forced) to visit a dying loved one or to attend the funeral services.

The grieving process is necessary to heal the wounds caused by the loss of someone dear to them. It helps one adjust to a new environment alone. The person will be able to withdraw their emotional energy and reinvest it in other relationships. When they can think of the deceased with sadness, and not wrenching pain, the grieving person is recovering. Though the loved one will never be forgotten, pleasant memories will replace the sad, painful ones.

Years later, if you listen to someone describe the loss of a cherished loved one, you may hear remnants of unresolved grief. They may think of the person all the time, may hold onto an old anger at someone, be unable to mention the loved one's name without tears, or may apologize repeatedly because of an imagined neglect.

Surviving a Personal Loss

Thirteen years passed before I was able to end my hidden, unresolved mourning. I owe the closure to an astute lady who commented, "You are the saddest person I have known." Of course I smiled and disagreed and she quietly asked if I knew how to say goodbye.

Although a nurse, I was not prepared to lose a husband, mother and son within a few years. A year after my 19-year-old son was diagnosed with cancer, my husband died unexpectedly. Several years later, with my newly-paralyzed son at home (waiting for admission to a rehabilitation center), I learned that my mother had died in a distant state. My son was admitted on an emergency basis. He was alone with strangers as I flew home to my grieving 82-year-old father. On the day following the funeral, I was informed that my son had a brain tumor. I left my father and returned to my son. When did I find time to mourn? A nurse remains calm and in control, and I did.

My son's death was unexpected, for in my denial, I accepted that his chronic condition was stable. With chemotherapy treatment and the remissions he had had, I was convinced that he would survive and continue his life. We were waiting for a new cure. During and following the funeral I was calm and supportive. I returned to work a week later. After a few days my heart began throwing frequent skipped beats (PVCs). The doctor prescribed sedation and told me to remain bedfast for a week. The heart arrhythmia has never returned. The stress from my loss had caught up with me.

The years went by, and except for sudden tears when I saw a tall, dark-haired young man with a mustache, it seemed my grief was past. I considered if I could have done more for my son, and wondered why I could not have saved him. My family's assurances that I was a devoted and resourceful mother did not seem to change my thoughts.

Then I was asked by a friend if I knew how to say good-bye and I realized that I did not. Although I was able to express my thoughts to my husband before his death, I had not had the same opportunity with my mother and son. My friend explained that there are many ways to say good-bye, but one symbolic way was to write a letter to your deceased loved ones. I could share my feelings and express my appreciation that they had been a part of my life for awhile. During the week I prepared to write the letters, I had actual physical pain and cried often. Gradually through the sad memories emerged a remembrance of happy times together. I had finally released my unexpressed grief, suffered the pain of my loss and found the meaning of our lives together.

In my letter, I told my son that he had been a wonderful gift to me and how much I loved him. I remembered our happy times, then I told him it was time to say goodbye and that we would meet again. I wrote a similar letter to my mother. Although I had to stop writing at times, because I could not see the paper through my tears, the feelings expressed in each letter wiped out my pain. I forgave myself for my imperfections and was thankful for the years we had shared.

I shared the letters with my sister and then carefully tore them into small pieces. I had finally had the talks with my loved ones that I had been denied. The dark cloud of loss and sadness that had overshadowed my daily life disappeared. I began to recall funny, happy moments that I had forgotten, and I always smile when I think of them today. It had taken thirteen years to heal.

> *Sometimes we think the pattern for the tapestry*
> *of our lives must have gotten lost.*
> *At those times we must stop and listen*
> *to the sound of the weaving that still goes on.*
> *Gail Kittleson wrote on a*
> *card from "The Sometimes Line"*

Resources for Caregivers

When I decided to write this book, I visited libraries in many states, built a small personal library and ask questions of everyone. I discovered that a large city library system has the budget to purchase a wide selection of reading materials, but small-town librarians must use great care in stretching their funds for community enrichment. Several of my recommendations were found in small city libraries.

The Inter-library Loan System

If you do not find the books you need, use the free library-to-library loan system. Many libraries are connected by a data base or you may complete the national loan form. You may wait for 1-3 weeks if the book is located within the state, and up to six months if the search reaches out of state. Through this service all books are available to everyone, everywhere. Ask the librarian for assistance.

Here is a list of sources that may help you find solutions to your problems:

Comprehensive Cancer Centers

A comprehensive cancer center (research and treatment) is located in most states. Listed are the name and location of each center.

Alabama — University of Alabama Cancer Center, Birmingham
Arizona — University of Arizona, School of Medicine, Tucson
California — Kenneth Norris Jr. Cancer Center, USC, Los Angeles
Connecticut — Yale School of Medicine, New Haven,
District of Columbia — Lombardi Cancer Research Center,
Washington D.C.
Florida — Sylvester Cancer Center, University of Miami, Miami
Maryland — John Hopkins Oncology Center, Baltimore
Massachusetts — Dana-Farber Cancer Institute, Boston
Michigan — University of Michigan Cancer Center, Detroit
Minnesota — Mayo Comprehensive Cancer Center, Rochester

New Hampshire — Norris Cotton Center, Dartmouth-Hitchcock
            Medical Center, Hanover
New York — Memorial Sloan-Kettering Cancer Center, New York
            Roswell Park Cancer Institute, Buffalo
            Columbia University Cancer Center,
              College of Physicians, New York
            New York University Medical Center, New York
North Carolina — Duke Cancer Center, Durham
            Lineberger Cancer Center, University of North
              Carolina School of Medicine, Chapel Hill
            Wake Forest University Cancer Center,
              Bowman Gray School of Medicine,
              Winston-Salem
Ohio — Ohio State University, Authur G. James Cancer
            Hospital, Columbus
Pennsylvania — Fox Chase Cancer Center, Philadelphia
            University of Pennsylvania Cancer Center,
              Philadelphia
            University of Pittsburgh Cancer Institute,
              Pittsburgh
Texas — University of Texas, M. D. Anderson Cancer Center,
            Houston
Vermont — University of Vermont, Vermont Regional Cancer
            Center, Burlington
Washington — Fred Hutchinson Cancer Center, Seattle
Wisconsin — University of Wisconsin Cancer Center, Madison

Health Hot Lines

1. National Information System for Health-Related Services.
    1-800-922-9234 (9-5 EST, weekdays)
    Information about specialized services for children with disabili-
    ties. Will refer to support groups, diagnostic & treatment centers
    across the U.S.

2. American Foundation for the Blind.
1-800-232-5463 (8:30-4:30 EST, weekdays)
News of the latest products for the blind. Information on vision loss, blindness, and services available to the blind. Will send free brochures.

3. National Institute of Neurological Disorders and Stroke.
1-800-352-9424. (8:30-5 EST, weekdays)
Information packets on neurological disorders including stroke, epilepsy, Parkinson's disease and spinal injuries. You can request referrals to support groups and other organizations.

4. National Mental Health Association.
1-800-969-6642 (9-5 EST, weekdays, recording other times)
Brochures on stress, depression, schizophrenia and other mental health problems. Will send a list of local organizations.

5. American Amputee Foundation.
1-800-553-4483 (8:30-5 EST, weekdays)
An information clearinghouse provides information and referral services designed to answer questions concerning the needs of amputees and those confined to wheelchairs.

6. US Department of Health and Human Services - MEDICARE.
1-800-368-5779 (Available 24 hours a day)
Answers questions about Medicare coverage; handles complaints on evidence of fraud or abuse in Medicare and Medicaid programs.

7. Arthritis Medical Center.
1-800-327-3027 (9-3 EST, weekdays)
Sends information on the Holistic Approach to the treatment of arthritis.

8. Asthma-Lung Disease Hotline.
1-800-222-LUNG (8-5 EST, weekdays)
Answers questions about asthma, emphysema, chronic bronchitis, tuberculosis, and environmental lung diseases. R.N.s and other health professionals answer questions.

9. Dial-a-Hearing Screening Test.
    1-800-222-EARS (9-6 EST, weekdays)
    Tells where to call in your area for a free hearing screening test.
    Offers numbers for self-help groups.

10. AIDS Hotline.
     1-800-342-AIDS, (in Spanish) 1-800-342-SIDA (24 hours a day)
     Recorded message explains symptoms, means of transmission and
     high-risk categories; gives address for brochure "Facts About Aids"
     and other publications.

11. ALANON Family Group.
     1-800-356-9996 (24 hrs. a day)
     Provides information about alcoholism specifically aimed at the
     families of alcoholics. Referral to local chapters.

12. American Institute for Preventative Medicine.
     1-800-345-AIPM (8:30-4:30 weekdays)
     Provides information about programs to stop smoking, reduce
     stress, control weight and other issues of health education.

13. American Parkinson's Disease Association.
     1-800-223-2732 (8:30-5 weekdays)
     Sends brochures, offers information on medicines combatting
     Parkinson's Disease, and provides referrals.

14. Epilepsy Foundation of America.
     1-800-332-1000 (9-5 EST weekdays)
     Provides assistance and counseling for epileptic patients and their
     families. Will send information on request.

15. Hill-Burton Free Hospital Care.
     1-800-638-0742 (9:30-5:30 EST weekdays)
     Sponsored by the Department of Health and Human Services.
     Sends information to callers about free care in hospitals and other
     health facilities, including a list of facilities in the caller's local area
     that participate in the program. The caller will be advised about
     how to file a complaint about the program. Service is primarily for

low-income people without Medicare or Medicaid to cover the costs of medical care.

16. Second Opinion Hotline for Non-Emergency Surgery.
    1-800-638-6833 (8-12 EST seven days a week)
    A project of the Health-Care Finance Administration; provides free referrals to specialists to double-check advice before an operation (fee for second opinion may be covered by insurance).

17. The Living Bank.
    1-800-528-2971 (24 hours a day, everyday)
    Information and registry for people to donate their organs, tissues, bones, or bodies for transplant or research.

Consumer Hotlines

1. Civil Rights Hotline.
   1-800-368-1019 (9-5:50 EST M-F)
   Accepts calls regarding discrimination on the basis of race, color, national origin, handicap or age occurring in Health and Human Services programs; e.g. in-admission, service or access to hospitals, nursing homes, day care centers or state health care assistance.

2. Fair Housing and Equal Opportunity Hotline.
   1-800-424-8590 (9-5 EST M-F)
   A project of Dept. of Housing and Urban Development. Accepts complaints of discrimination in housing based on race, color, religion, sex, national origin, family status or handicap.

3. Higher Education/Adult Training for People with
    Handicaps (HEATH).
   1-800-544-3284 (8:45-4:45 EST M-F)
   Sponsored by the American Council on Education. Offers information about post-secondary education options open to handicapped individuals.

4. National Tour Association-Handicapped Travel Division.
    1-800-NTA-8886 (8-5 EST M-F)
    Provides a list of member tour operators who specialize in travel services to handicapped individuals, guaranteeing access busses, hotel rooms and destinations.

5. Tele-Consumer Hotline.
    1-800-332-1124 (9-5 EST M-F)
    Answers questions on long-distance options and service, telephone equipment and repairs, ways to cut costs, and where to get help resolving billing problems.

Other Information Sources

Sensory Stimulation Products (Alzheimer's Disease, Dementia).

The company specializes in caregiving resources for Alzheimer's and other persons with dementia. They have over 450 products for stimulating sensory awareness, making daily living activities easier and offering comfort and nurturing. Many are multi-dimensional and adapt to different cognitive levels. The catalogue includes a Deterioration Scale to help the caregiver assess the level of degeneration. You may request the product catalogue or education catalogue (or both). Write to Geriatric Resources, P.O. Box 1509, Goldenrod, FL, 32733-1509. Phone 1-800-359-0309 or (407) 678-1616.

Hints for the Disabled.

Patricia Galbreaith has written an informative column for a number of years, titled "Hints for the Disabled." She is an excellent resource for difficult-to-find sources for assistance. In a recent column she listed where to get the latest research information on Scleroderma, a resource directory for amputees, and an agency to contact if you are a victim of fraud. Address your letters to Patricia Galbreaith, The Dallas Morning News, P.O. Box 268, Weatherford, TX, 76086.

Medical Supplies.

The time spent on comparison shopping may save money. Write for medical supply and medical warehouse catalogues and compare their prices with local medical equipment and supply stores. You may ask if small quantities are available. Two examples are: Medical Line Warehouse, 6130 Clark Center Ave. # 103, Sarasota, FL, 34238. Phone 1-800-247-2256
St. Louis Medical Supply, 10821 Manchester Rd.at Lindbergh Blvd. Kirkwood, MO, 63122. Phone 1-800-950-6020 or (314) 821-7355

Wheelchair Product Report.

AARP has prepared a 10-page report on the wheelchairs available. It is based on a study of 19 wheelchairs where users tested and rated the chairs based on different tasks. Write to Wheelchair Report (D14049), AARP Fulfillment (EEO118), 1909 D. Street, N.W. Washington D.C. 20049. Allow 6-8 weeks for delivery.

HIV Drug Service.

On July 23, 1995, a non-profit group launched a mail-order prescription drug service to provide medicines for anyone with HIV or AIDS at discount prices and with complete confidentiality. MedExpress service will provide drugs, vitamins and nutrients at 25-30% less than commercial mail-order pharmacies. Customers may call MedExpress, 1-800-808-8060 to place orders which will be delivered 24 to 48 hours later by Airborne Express. The shipment arrives in a non-descript secure package. MedExpress will handle all types of payments; Medicaid, private insurance, etc.

The Technical Aid Project.

The Tetra Development Society has a project in which a person with severe disabilities can get help in developing assistive devices not available commercially. It brings together the person with a need and the technical people, such as engineers and manufacturers, who volunteer their time to design and produce a suitable device. They will also adapt existing devices to meet the needs of the disabled person. You may address a letter to Pat Blackburn, Project Coordinator, Tetra Development Society, Plaza of Nations, Box 27, 770 Pacific Boulevard South, Vancouver, British Columbia V6B 5E7, Canada.

Make Today Count, Inc.

The local chapters of the organization provide information and emotional support to people with life-threatening diseases and their caregivers. They publish a bi-monthly newsletter that offers tips on caregiving and inspirational reading. Workshops and seminars are one of their projects. Local chapters offer volunteer-based services such as group meetings, a telephone "buddy" system, home and hospital visits and emergency transportation. You may call or write the national office to locate the chapter near you or send $1.00 for a copy of the national registry of local chapters. Write to Make Today Count, Inc., 101 1/2 South Union Station, Alexandria, VA 22314-3323. Phone 215/ 945-6900.

The Sometimes Line

Gail Kittleson has produced a line of cards whose verses express the unspoken feelings of caregivers and friends during moments of pain and loss. You may write to "The Sometimes Line," P.O. Box 638, Greene, IA, 50636 for information and illustrations of her beautifully written words.

Sources for Assistance

Project LINK

A free information service established by the Center for Therapeutic Applications of Technology (University of Buffalo), helps people learn about assistive devices. Users are asked to answer a few questions about their condition and the activities that pose the most difficulty for them. The service will select and send catalogs and brochures for products related to their needs. By compiling a national, confidential database of people with disabilities and linking them with companies that make the products, the LINK project helps bring the two groups together. Contact Sherry Altman, Coordinator, Project LINK, CTAT/UB, 525 Kimball Tower, Buffalo, NY 14214. Phone: 1-800-628-2281 or (716) 829-3141.

ABLEDATA

A national database of information for over 18,000 products for people with disabilities (including price and company information) has an information specialist to answer questions and provide referrals free of charge. ABLEDATA can be searched for different models of a specific device. Call or write NARIC's Information Team at 8455 Colesville Road, Suite 935, Silver Spring, MD, 20910, Phone: 1-800-227-0216 or (301) 588-9284 (both numbers Voice/TDD)

The Doable, Renewable Home

This free 36-page booklet (Pub. No. D12470) is available from AARP. It explains design concepts and products that help make homes more comfortable for people who experience physical limitations. The book lists publications that give helpful advice on adapting a home and names the manufacturers of these products. Write AARP Fulfillment, 601 E Street, NW, Washington, DC 20049

The National Accessible Apartment Clearinghouse [NAAC]

A service developed by the National Apartment Association offers help to people with disabilities searching for suitable housing. It provides an updated list of existing units in your area, the addresses, features that make the units accessible and how they are managed. The list is available free of charge by calling 1-800-421-1221 for a copy. Not included are those listed under Section Eight of the Housing Authority. (From Patricia Galbreaith's Column, "Hints for the Disabled")

Resource Directory for Older People

Prepared by the National Institute on Aging, the directory lists 200 national organizations that offer social services, consumer advice, health information, legal aid, etc. for older Americans and their families. Included in the list are federal agencies, professional societies, private groups and voluntary programs, with a brief description of each group and the service it provides. To receive one free copy of the 224 page directory, write to NIA Information Center: Directory, P.O. Box 8057, Gaithersburg, MD 20898-8057.

Source for Needed Medications

The research-based pharmaceutical industry has had a long-standing tradition of providing prescription medicines free of charge to physicians whose patients might not otherwise have access to the necessary medicines. Each of the 63 companies base the patient's eligibility on a different criteria; from having exhausted all Medicaid, Medicare, third-party insurance and social agencies to an eligibility based on an annual income. Most large pharmaceutical companies participate in this plan to provide needed medications for those who have little money to pay for them. Doctors must recommend patients for the program by contacting the company directly. For a copy of "Program to Help Older Americans Obtain Their Medications," write The Senate Committee on Aging Publications, U.S. Senate, Washington, DC 20510-6400.

Source for Emergency Funds for Alzheimer's Families

The American Health Assistance Foundation has funded a family relief program. The Alzheimer's patient and his family caregivers can receive a grant of up to $500 for emergency expenses, when other means of paying for care and treatment have been depleted. Expenses may be for nursing and respite care, day services, medications and medical supplies, transportation, living expenses or other costs related to caring for someone with Alzheimer's. For information on how to apply, contact Jean Butts, program administrator, at 1-800-437-2423.

Resource for Eye Treatment

The National Eye Care Project is dedicated to the prevention of blindness. Anyone 65 years or older who needs surgery or medicine for their eyes, but cannot afford it, will be referred to an opthalmologist (an MD specializing in eye care) who can provide care at no out-of pocket expense. They can also help the person to draw on Medicaid, Medicare, insurance or the divisions of blind services (third-party payers.) Call 1-800-222-EYES.

Veterans Benefits

Seven million World War II veterans are over 65 today and by 1999 the total number will increase to 37% of the veteran population. The VA health care system is revamping its programs to meet the complex needs of an aging constituency. The updated 1994 edition of "Federal Benefits for Veterans and Dependents" includes the eligibility guidelines, claims procedures, a list of addresses and phone numbers of all VA offices, medical centers, etc.

You may order a copy from the U.S. Government Printing Office, Superintendent of Documents, P.O. Box 37194, Pittsburg, PA 15220-7954. Cost is $2.50 per copy.

Travel by the Disabled Person

Travel may be more difficult when one is disabled, but possible and enjoyable with planning, patience and determination. Find a sympathetic travel agent, then write the department of tourism or the Chamber of Commerce (city) where you plan to go and ask for guide booklets for the handicapped.

For travel information, write to The Society for the Advancement of Travel for the Handicapped, Penthouse Suite, 26 Court Street, Brook- lyn, N.Y. 11242. Whole Person Tours publishes *The Itinerary: The Magazine for Travelers with Physical Disabilities*, P.O. Box 1084, Bayonne, NJ 07002

Book and Magazines Designed for Those with Disabilities

Several informative magazines are available for those living with disabilities. An excellent example is the quarterly magazine, "Accent On Living" which combines articles from the disabled or their families with descriptions and pictures of new products. The address is: Accent on Living, PO Box 700, Bloomington, Illinois, 61702. Cost is $10.00 per year.

Other publications such as Paraplegic News (official magazine from the Paralyzed Veterans of America), The Squeaky Wheel (from the National Paraplegia Foundation) and Performance (by President's Committee on Employment of the Handicapped) are available. Check with the research department in the public library for addresses and phone numbers.

The book, *Safe Use of Medicines by Older People*, published by the National Institute on Aging, is currently available in English and Chinese. This book is being translated into Spanish also. To order write to the National Institute on Aging Information Center, P.O. Box 8057, Gaitherburg, MD 20898-8057

Products that Help the Disabled Person

Braille or Large-Type Overlays

Overlays for the control panels or dials for major appliances are offered by these manufacturers:

1. General Electric provides knobs free of charge for any GE or Hotpoint range and panels for the laundry equipment. Send the model and serial numbers to GE Consumer Affairs, GE Appliances, AP6-106 Appliance Park, Louisville, KY, 40225

2. Whirlpool Appliance Group offers the same products as well as Braille or audio-cassette manuals. These overlays can be requested from the dealer when the appliance is purchased or call Whirlpool's Consumer Assistance Center. Phone - 800-253-1301, or 800-253-1121 (from Hawaii)

3. Sears offers a braille kit which includes the same products and may be ordered when a microwave is purchased.

4. Maytag Company does not (but suggests using a labeling machine to make your own.)

5. A touchable phone attachment with oversized numbers will clamp over the push buttons on any standard phone. If you cannot find one locally, call 1-800-323-5547 for the Enrichment catalogue.

Tips to Make a Home Safer and More Accessible

1. Replace the outside door with an extra-wide 34-inch door to allow a wheelchair easy access.

2. A low-pile carpet provides a slip-free surface for wheelchairs.

3. Remove coffee tables and scatter rugs if someone uses a walker or has impaired vision.

4. Place a lever type door knob extender (about $13-15) over a round doorknob. If you cannot find one locally, call 1-800-323-5547 for their Enrichments catalogue.

5. Put a 150-200 watt bulb in a lamp and use a lamp dimmer switch ($13.-15.) to adjust the light in the room. Search for small lights that come on when doors are opened ($8.-10.) to put in closets, cabinets etc. If you cannot find one, call 1-800- 342-9988 for their Solutions catalogue.

6. An L-shaped toilet paper holder ($15.-17.) makes changing roles easier. If you cannot find one, call 1-800-421-2961 for the Hafele Corporation.

7. Long handled barbeque tools are aids for wheelchair bound cooks. "Good Grip" kitchen tools (under $10. each) are available from Self Care catalogue (1-800-345-4021) and For Convenience Sake catalogue (1-800-242-9763.)

8. Place grab bars on the bathtub or on the wall next to tubs and toilets to prevent bathroom falls. If you don't find ones you like, call Tubular Specialties (1-800-421-2961) or Franklin Brass Manufacturing (1-800-421-3375) for catalogues.

9. Move the electrical outlet plugs 25 inches above the floor.

Note: Check the library for product catalogues or write for the *Access with Ease* 1993, a catalogue of products to make life easier. Write Access with Ease, Inc. P.O.Box 1150, Chino Valley, AZ 86323. Phone: 602-636-9469.

(From "A Houseful of Ideas for Safe Living", *Aging Magazine*, 1994.)

Talking Books Programs For The Blind

1. Recordings for the Blind.   Dept. N81, 215 E. 58th St.
   Has 50,000 text books   New York, NY 10022.
   To apply for membership: Phone (212)751-0860

2. Volunteer Services.   Dept. N81, 814 W. Wisconsin Ave.
   If they don't have a book   Milwaukee, WS 53233
   on tape, they will tape on   Phone (414)278-3039
   request (free if returned in one
   year, if kept, charge is $2.00).

3. Library for the Blind.   Library for the Blind and
   Located in every state   Physically Handicapped
   Will also record on request.   919 Walnut St.
                                     Philadelphia, PA. 19107

Shots and Vaccines

1. A pneumococcal vaccine which prevents the type of bacterial
pneumonia that kills thousands of people each year is available.
People who are 65 years of age or older and those who have a
chronic illness or a weakened immune system are encouraged to get
the one-shot protection. Those over 65 are three times more likely to
get the bacterial pneumonia (as distinguished from viral) than the
general public. It is a disease that can be fatal. The vaccine prevents
88% of the bacteria that cause pneumonia. Most people need to get
the shot only once; however, some older people may need a booster
shot. Check with your doctor. The shot is covered by Medicare.

2. Medicare will pay for flu shots and will reimburse the cost of
therapeutic shoes for diabetics. The addition of these benefits is
based on research that has shown that flu shots will cut down on
hospitalizations from pneumonia.

Index

Bibliography/Recommended Reading

Caring for the Caregiver

MAINSTAY: FOR THE WELL SPOUSE OF THE CHRONICALLY ILL
by Maggie Strong, Little Brown & Co., New York, 1988.

TAKING CARE OF THE CAREGIVER by Jeannie D. Roberts
Palo Alto, CA., Bull Publishing, 1991.

WHEN A LOVED ONE IS ILL by Leonard Felder, Ph.D.
New York, New American Library, 1990.

Doctor-Patient-Caregiver Relationship

HOW TO TALK TO YOUR DOCTOR by Janet R. Maurer, M.D.
New York, Simon & Schuster, 1986

PARENTCARE by Lissy Jarvik, M.D.,Ph.D. and Garry Small, M.D.
New York, Bantam Books, 1988

WE ARE NOT ALONE by Sephra Kobrin Pitzele
New York, Workman Publishing, 1986

Caring for a Disabled Loved One

EXTENDED HEALTH CARE AT HOME by Evelyn M. Baulch
Berkeley, CA, Celestial Arts, 1988

HOME CARE FOR THE ELDERLY by Jay Portnow, M.D. and
Martha Houtmann R.N., New York, Pocket Books, 1987

REACH FOR FITNESS by Richard Simmons
New York, Warners Books, 1986

THE CAREGIVER'S GUIDE by Carolyn Rob, R.N. and Janet
Reynolds G.N.P.
Boston, MS, Houghton Miffin, 1991

Meeting the Body's Needs

FOOD - YOUR MIRACLE MEDICINE by Jean Carter
New York, Harper-Collins, 1993

Helping With Mobility

GETTING BACK ON YOUR FEET by Sally R. Pryor
Post Hills, VT, Chelsea Green Publishing, 1991

Cancer

A CANCER PATIENT'S GUIDE TO RADIATION THERAPY by
Richard A Steeves, Madison, WI, Medical Physics Publishing,
1992

COPING WITH CHEMOTHERAPY by Nancy Bruning
Garden City, NY, The Dial Press, 1985

LOVE, MEDICINE & MIRACLES by Bernie S. Siegel, M.D.
New York, Harper & Row, 1986

Stroke

AFTER THE STROKE by Evelyn Urban Shirk
Buffalo, NY, Prometheus Books, 1991

STROKES: WHAT FAMILIES SHOULD KNOW by Elaine
Fantle Shimbery, New York, Ballantine Books, 1990

Alzheimer's Disease

ALZHEIMER'S by Howard Gruetzner, M.Ed.
New York, John Wiley & Sons, 1992

CARING FOR THE ALZHEIMER'S PATIENT by
Raye Lynne Dipple, Ph.D. and J. Thomas Hutton, M.D. Ph.D.
New York, Prometheus Books, 1988

Chronic Conditions That Influence Caregiving

ADDICTIVE DRINKING by Clark Vaughn
   New York, Viking Press, 1982

FAMILY MATTERS by Daniel Gottlieb, Ph.D. and Edward Claflin
   New York, Penguin Books, 1991

HOW TO LIVE WITH A NEUROTIC by Albert Ellis, PH.D.
   CA, General Publishing, 1975, Copyrighted by the Institute
For Rational — Emotive Therapy

When You Can No Longer Provide Alone

ELDERCARE: CHOOSING AND FINANCING LONG TERM CARE
   by Joseph Matthews, Berkley, CA, Nolo Press, 1990

HOW TO CHOOSE A NURSING HOME by Joanne
   Meshinsky, R.N., New York, Avon Books, 1991

NURSING HOME HANDBOOK by Jo Horne
   Glenview, IL, AARP Books, 1989

VALIDATION: HOW TO HELP DISORIENTED OLD-OLD by
   Naomi Feil, ACSW, Cleveland, OH, Edward Feil Productions,
1989

When a Loved One's Life is Ending

DEATH: THE FINAL STAGE OF GROWTH by
   Elizabeth Kuebler-Ross, M.D., New York, Simon &
   Schuster, 1986

LIVING WITH DYING by David Carroll
   New York, McGraw Hill, 1985

Articles - Medical Journals and Magazines

1. "Troubleshooting Ostomy Problems" by Mildred G. Kemp, RN, Ph.D. GERIATRIC NURSING, September/October, 1990, pp. 233-236.

2. "Helping Ostomy Patients Manage Medications" by Michelle A. Madda, R.N.,C.,B.S.N., NURSING 91, March, 1991, pp. 47-49.

3. OSTOMY QUARTERLY MAGAZINE, United Ostomy Association, Inc. Irvine, CA.

4. "Controlling Adverse Effects of Chemotherapy" by Dawn Camp-Sorrell, R.N., O.C.N., M.S.N., NURSING 91, April, 1991, pp. 34-41.

5. "Seeing Through the Mask of Cancer" by Janet Spindler, R.N. NURSING 91, May, 1991. pp. 37-40.

6. "Guidelines for Treatment of Cancer Pain" by Texas Cancer Council, Austin, Texas, 1991

7. "Understanding Your Grief" by St. Anthony's Hospice, Amarillo, Texas, 1989

8. "Understanding the Final Messages of the Dying" by Maggie Pflaum Callahan, R.N. and Patricia Kelley, R.N., NURSING 86, June, 1986, pp. 26-30.

9. THE AGING MAGAZINE, published annually by the Administration on Aging in the Department of Health, Education and Welfare.

10. "The Lowest-Tech Medicine Ever" by Gurney Williams, LONGEVITY MAGAZINE, January, 1992, pp. 60-69.

Order Form

COPING WITH CAREGIVING: A Common-Sense Approach to Home Care is a book with hundreds of tips and shortcuts for the busy home caregiver.

If you cannot find COPING WITH CAREGIVING at your local stores, order directly from Ruhl Press. Fill out the order form below and return with your check or money order to:

RUHL PRESS
P.O. Box 8100-153
Amarillo, TX 79114

Remember, the book makes a great gift for the home caregiver.

COPING WITH CARGIVING ______ copy	$14.95 each	______
Additional ______ copies	$12.95 each	______
Postage/Handling	Add $3.00/one copy	______
Additional copies	Add $2.00/each additional	______
Texas residents	Add $1.22/each sales tax	______
	TOTAL	______

Print or Type

Name ____

Address _____________________________________

____

City _________________ State _________ Zip ________

Quantity discounts are available on bulk purchases of this book for workshops, fund raising or gift giving. Special booklets can be created to fit your special needs. For information contact Ruhl Press, P.O. Box 8100-153, Amarillo, Texas 79114, Phone or Fax 806-354-8248.